ACIDOPHILUS

AND

COLON
HEALTH

BOOK YOUR PLACE ON OUR WEBSITE AND MAKE THE READING CONNECTION!

We've created a customized website just for our very special readers, where you can get the inside scoop on everything that's going on with Zebra, Pinnacle and Kensington books.

When you come online, you'll have the exciting opportunity to:

- View covers of upcoming books
- Read sample chapters
- Learn about our future publishing schedule (listed by publication month *and author*)
- Find out when your favorite authors will be visiting a city near you
- Search for and order backlist books from our online catalog
- Check out author bios and background information
- Send e-mail to your favorite authors
- Meet the Kensington staff online
- Join us in weekly chats with authors, readers and other guests
- Get writing guidelines
- AND MUCH MORE!

**Visit our website at
http://www.kensingtonbooks.com**

ACIDOPHILUS
AND
COLON
HEALTH

■

THE NATURAL WAY
TO PREVENT DISEASE

David Webster

KENSINGTON BOOKS
Kensington Publishing Corp.
http://www.kensingtonbooks.com

This publication and product is designed to provide accurate and authoritative information with regard to the subject matter covered. The purchase of this publication does not create a doctor-patient relationship between the purchaser and the author, nor should the information contained in this book be considered specific medical advice with respect to a specific patient and/or a specific condition. In the event the purchaser desires to obtain specific medical advice or other information concerning a specific person, condition, or situation, the services of a competent professional should be sought.

The author and publisher specifically disclaim any liability, loss, or risk, personal or otherwise, that is or may be incurred as a consequence, directly or indirectly, of the use and application of any of the information contained in this book.

KENSINGTON BOOKS are published by

Kensington Publishing Corp.
850 Third Avenue
New York, NY 10022

Copyright © 1999 by David Webster

First Trade Printing: October, 1999
First Paperback Printing: October, 2000
10 9 8 7 6 5 4 3 2 1

Printed in the United States of America

ACKNOWLEDGMENTS

My heartfelt gratitude to Suzanne E. Sky. Her guidance, research, editing, writing, and support of my work over the past twenty years made this book possible.

To Richard Renn, D.O., without whose help this work would not have been realized today.

To Francis Gibson, D.C., who inspired me.

To Mr. Fritz, who handed me Dr. Empringham's manuscript, which was the driving force behind my work.

To Mr. Max, our springer spaniel, who helped with his great spirit for eleven years.

Special thanks to everyone who has helped bring this book to fruition: You know who you are.

PERMISSIONS

Book Illustrations:

CONTENTS

(Gas-Forming Foods • Dry Foods and Fiber • Alcohol • High-Protein, High-Fat Diets • Raw Protein Foods • Remedy for Problem Foods) • Enjoy Life! • Questions and Answers

FOREWORD

■

I first met David Webster in 1979 in Hawaii, where he shared the full scope of his work with me. I received a copy of his booklet, *Acidophilus & Colon Health*, and immediately called him to learn more. As a busy osteopathic doctor, I realized his knowledge about the colon flora was the missing link necessary to achieve a lasting foundation of health and immunity. Together, David and I set up the initial protocol for the procedure now known as the Webster Implant Technique™. Working together, we did a test study with my patients and I found that over a third of my most difficult cases quickly recovered their health after following David's program. This encouraged and inspired David to continue his work and research in California, where he has provided his successful Webster Implant Technique™ in Encinitas since 1991.

David is the first to explain so clearly how the colon is a key component of the immune system and how maintaining the colon in its natural acidic state is essential for a healthy liver, bloodstream, and physical health. Best of all, David's methods work. His procedure is excellent when used as part of an overall program to restore health.

I would suggest David's protocol as a starting place when a person has elimination difficulties or any chronic health problem. It is helpful and essential for people of all constitutions, whether they are weak or strong, because it cleanses and nourishes the person at the same time and very quickly helps to restore colon health in most cases. We all know that if the major organs of elimination are not working properly, a person cannot achieve or maintain good health. Once the colon is cleared and its natural acidic acidophilus flora is restored, we can then do deeper work to clear and heal the whole person. A follow-up treatment with David's protocol is also advisable when a person is on the road to recovery. Since a healthy acidophilus colon flora is the foundation of good health, this reinforces the healing work already done and allows the body to heal more deeply with lasting results.

David has made a substantial contribution to current medical knowledge. He gives us the key to keeping our immune system intact as we face the current threats of bacterial and other illnesses. By applying the knowledge in this book to your daily life, you can reclaim the health that is your birthright and reap the benefits of lasting health.

Richard Renn, D.O.

PREFACE

■

"Balance is the Law, Purification the Goal." These summarize my intent from the beginning. In order to be in balance with natural laws, however, we need to apply our knowledge to the task, and especially the scientific knowledge presented here. Look around you: Toxic conditions are increasing daily. And the more toxins you take into your body without doing anything about it, the more you will suffer their effects. For example, if your colon is alkaline due to secretions from pathogens harbored there, toxins and their insidious by-products are already building up. They are like termites eating away at your foundation without your realizing it. If the floor suddenly breaks one day due to deterioration, it may be too late to repair it. To have a strong floor, to fight deterioration by insects, you must protect it—and the same goes for your body. To have a good, strong immune system, the colon and bloodstream must be as clean as possible. So start now and cleanse your system, cleanse it as you would clean anything to preserve its longevity, but do so wisely and by virtue of what you will read in this book.

We are paying with our health and bank account for conditions that develop in the colon; we are paying even more because scientific replacement of acidophilus is still not an established medical procedure. Yeast infections, irritable bowel syndrome (IBS), and other chronic conditions could be eliminated in a short time by restoring the healthy colon acidophilus correctly as the foundation for health.

With this book, you now possess a manual to build your health from the foundation up. Everyone who wants to can benefit from the simple facts presented here. Because the knowledge in this book is based on natural laws using natural substances, you can be confident of attaining lasting results to improve your health and longevity.

Everyone is unique in his or her genetics, constitution, and lifestyle. But basic principles of health can still be understood and applied for everyone's benefit. Today, with the wide use of alcohol, antibiotics, and medications along with constant exposure to air pollution, pesticides, preservatives, and stress, it is imperative that we create and maintain a healthy colon and immune system. We must live in balance with all organisms, and good health allows us to do so.

It has been well over twenty years since I set foot on this path. My work is based on scientific principles that were first well established in Europe in the early 1900s, but which were discarded when antibiotics took center stage in the 1940s. Simply, those students who went to medical school after 1940 lost out. They were not taught the basics of colon health, of how the colon with an alkaline pH is the root cause of degenerative disease.

The fathers of medicine have well established that everyone is genetically unique, and that, just as water flows to the lowest point in the valley, toxins in the bloodstream flow to the weakest points in the body. Even Louis Pasteur, the scientist who first found that bacteria cause infection, did not fully understand the implications here. His brilliant colleague, the scientist Pierre Bechamp, tried to point out to Pasteur that it was a mistake to fight and destroy pathogens in their own medium, where they proliferated best. Rather, the key lay in changing the medium.

Unfortunately, Bechamp's insight fell on deaf ears. Today's medical model follows Pasteur's approach of "search and destroy." This is why we are told we must "fight" all sorts of infections and diseases and, in the process, hopefully "win the battle" against them. Meanwhile, are we winning or are the microbes winning? Bacteria and viruses are mutating at an amazing rate, becoming resistant to many drugs and antibiotics. Medical science is running out of effective antibiotics with which to attack and kill them. In the long run, if we don't change our approach on a planetary scale, it will probably be the microbes, not humans, who will win this self-proclaimed war. Moreover, microbes have been here from the beginning of the earth and are an integral part of the cycles of life and death. How can we continue to survive as a species if, in fact, we do find a way to extinguish them entirely?

Years ago, when disease was spread by massive mosquito infestations, scientists finally realized the truth: to eradicate mosquito-borne illnesses, eliminate the stagnant water in which the mosquitoes bred. And the same principle holds for the colon. Changing the medium in the colon to a slightly acid pH—so that acidophilus flora will flourish and the pathogenic bacteria can no longer thrive—is the solution to many health problems. Just how can this be done? This information is the missing link in contemporary medical knowledge that I can give you.

A healthy colon flora provides the foundation for good health, immunity, and longevity. This is our birthright, a bacterial gift from nature. In this century, many factors have undermined this birthright. There is a simple and direct path that leads to health. Reading this book can be the first step on such a journey.

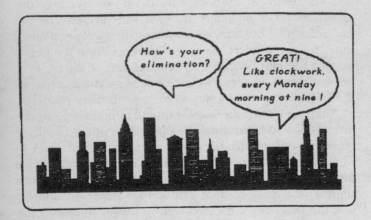

INTRODUCTION

For thousands of years, traditional medical practitioners have recognized the colon's influence on our immune system, health, and longevity. Since the beginning of recorded history, cultures across the globe have included specific methods for colon care in their health practices. With the upsurge of modern medical practices in the twentieth century, this knowledge has fallen by the wayside. Researchers who value the medical wisdom of older cultures, however, have rediscovered what was and will again be known about colon health and its relation to the body.

Humans have always instinctively felt the colon was a source of disease. Enemas as a medical practice were documented as far back as 5,000 years ago, again in cultures across the globe. These early practitioners also used a wide range of herbs to address and cleanse the colon as a means to health.

Today, science knows the colon as much more than an organ of elimination. It plays an important role as part of our immune system and in absorption of nutrients into the body. It influences liver, brain, and nerve function, and directly affects the function of other organs of elimination such as the kidneys, urinary bladder, lungs, and skin. The health of our colon determines the health of our bloodstream, organs, and tissues, thus also affecting our immunity and longevity.

Specifically, it is the bacteria inhabiting the colon that determines the health of the body directly and indirectly. In an adult, the beneficial colon flora consists of several species of bacteria, the two most important being *Lactobacillus acidophilus* and *Bifidobacterium bifidum*. What all acidophilus colon flora have in common, though, is their capacity to convert carbohydrates, specifically lactose (milk sugar) into lactic, acetic, and other slightly acidic by-products through a process of fermentation.

These bacteria can live only in a slightly acid environment. In Greek, the word "acidophilus" means "acid-loving." Since the families of acid-loving bacteria are very large, to simplify this text, all types of beneficial bacteria in the colon will hereafter be referred to as "acidophilus," unless referring to a specific species or type.

The acidophilus colon flora provides one of nature's first lines of defense in our bodies against invading microorganisms. When acidophilus are established in the healthy colon, disease-forming, opportunistic bacteria and other microorganisms are unable to take hold or survive. Thus, the acidophilus colon flora provides a protective shield.

Think of the colon as the soil of the body. The natural acidophilus colon flora are like flowers growing in healthy, well-balanced soil. Pathogens (disease-producing microorganisms) are like weeds that spread without limit in unhealthy soil.

The types of bacteria found in the colon can be grouped into two main categories, based on their metabolic by-products and effect on the host. Usually they are referred to as "good" or "bad" bacteria. "Bad" types of bacteria produce toxic by-products that contribute to long-term illness and chronic degeneration in the body. A "pathogen" is a microorganism or substance capable of producing disease.[1] Because of this, we will refer to this type of flora or bacteria as "pathogenic" because it is disease-causing.

The "good" acidophilus bacteria have a mutually supportive or symbiotic relationship with humans. We provide them with a place to live and they provide their beneficial by-products which acidify the colon, protect us against harmful, invasive bacteria or other pathogens, and produce specific nutrients which are utilized by our bodies. Because of their role, we refer to acidophilus as a "protective" or "beneficial" flora or bacteria.

These terms originated in the early days of research and are important tools to help simplify and understand the process occurring in the colon which influence our health, immunity, and longevity.

1

THE FATHERS OF COLON HEALTH

■

Two contexts inspired the research presented in this book: my personal experiences and the work of Dr. James Empringham and Professor Eli Metchnikoff. These two great scientists sought for ways to prolong life and improve immune function. And as they did so, they discovered that the true fountain of youth lies in our colon! Each man pioneered extensive research on the cause and relief of bacterial imbalance in the colon and on the importance of colon flora in health and disease. Their work laid the foundation on which modern researchers have expanded. Metchnikoff and Empringham found that acidophilus secretes slightly acid metabolic by-products that destroy or anesthetize pathogenic bacteria before they can take hold and cause disease in the body. They also found that the effect of bacterial secretions on human health is proportionate to their population size. When acidophilus predominate in the colon, pathogens can exist only in small numbers and their secretions are relatively harmless.

Eli Metchnikoff—Nobel Prize Winner

Metchnikoff's work provided the foundation for much of the microbiological and bacteriological scientific research done in the twentieth century. In fact, in 1895, he succeeded Pasteur as director of the Pasteur Institute and, in 1908, received the Nobel Prize for Medicine. Metchnikoff's research showed that pathogenic bacteria in the colon produce toxins that, when absorbed into the bloodstream, cause slow poisoning of the entire system. In one very large study, Metchnikoff analyzed fecal samples from patients all over France. Collaborating physicians supplied Metchnikoff with a patient history along with each sample. From this and his other studies, Metchnikoff was able to formulate six basic tenets, which are still important for us today.

1. There is a close correlation between a person's health and the type of bacteria that reside and predominate in their colon.
2. When the acidophilus flora is absent from the colon, the pathogenic bacteria dominates and secrete poisonous substances (toxins).
3. This formation of toxins can continue for many years before there is noticeable damage to an individual's health.
4. Each person will be affected differently by these toxins, depending on which organs or areas of their body are weak or vulnerable due to heredity or lifestyle. Some individuals will experience kidney disease, while others may experience prostate problems, breast cancer, headaches, allergies, or other illnesses.[1]

5. Toxins generated by the pathogenic colon flora enter the bloodstream and contribute to illness and degenerative disease.
6. The acidophilus colon flora provides the foundation of health in the body. It must be reestablished to prevent and alleviate disease and to promote health.

Metchnikoff was the first scientist to recognize the need for restoring the acidophilus flora as the fountain of health. Unfortunately, while he understood the microbiology at work here, his succeeding experiments were not as successful. To prove his point, he used a bovine strain of acidophilus, *L. bulgaricus,* that will not implant in the human colon under any circumstances. Only a human strain of acidophilus will implant in the human colon. His colleague, Dr. Empringham, and other modern scientists now understand what Metchnikoff needed for success. From Metchnikoff's failure we have gained an invaluable truth!

James Empringham

As a student of Metchnikoff's, Dr. James Empringham also did extensive fecal analysis and studies to determine what effect colon flora had on human health. A Doctor of Science and Regius Professor of Microbiology at St. Margaret's Hospital in London, Empringham also served as director of Kensington Laboratories for Scientific Research in London and lectured at the Physicians and Surgeons College of Microbiology. In 1926, he founded the Health Education Society in New York City, which offered inexpensive medical care and home visits by a staff of physicians and nurses who instructed people in health, hygiene, and disease prevention. What motivated Empringham? As a young man, he received a shattering diagnosis. He had a degenerative condition that would soon lead to his death.

Empringham well remembers his doctor's exact words: "You are an old man. Senility is not a question of the calendar—not a mere matter of the number of years since we came into the world. The degenerated condition of the body called 'old age' is merely a register of the damage that has been done to our organs and tissues by various poisons. You have the worst case of intestinal toxemia I have seen in a man of your years."[2]

At the same time Empringham received this diagnosis, Metchnikoff had just startled the scientific community by his discovery of the protective colon flora. Empringham lost no time. He left for the Pasteur Institute to learn all he could. By applying Metchnikoff's data on restoring the healthy colon acidophilus flora to his own condition, within one year Empringham found his health significantly improved. Having cheated the death diagnosed for him, he returned to England, where he continued his research on the acidophilus flora. By the way, his health steadily improved. Through his continuing research he corroborated the basic findings of Metchnikoff and then made some additional discoveries. His three most important discoveries were:

1. A human strain of acidophilus is the only strain that will establish itself in the human colon.
2. Acidophilus taken orally will not reestablish the protective colon flora.
3. A human strain of acidophilus must be implanted rectally for lasting results.

Through my research and experience, I have discovered alternative ways to replenish the natural colon flora that bring this field forward into the coming century.

Colon Hygiene

Hygiene derives from the Greek word meaning "healthful" with two secondary meanings: "clean" or "sanitary." Some seventy years ago, from the 1920s to the early 1930s, medical practitioners recognized the origin of many diseases in focal infections. As a result, their interest in colon hygiene was high. Focal infections, of course, were and are identified by three criteria: (1) they are located in one area of the body; (2) they take up residence there; and (3) they cause secondary infections in other areas of the body. At the time as well, their clinical experience told them that main sites for infection included the tonsils, nasal sinuses, gallbladder, appendix, roots of teeth, and, yes, the colon.[3] They well knew the colon, in fact, as an especially important site for focal infections—infections that led to disease in other areas of the body. Fortunately for us today, European doctors and many holistic professionals still consider focal infections, and the role of the colon in such infections, as a main cause of disease.

Capitalizing on the perspectives of his time, though, in 1923 Phillip Norman, M.D., invented a colonic gravity flow apparatus for implanting *L. acidophilus* rectally. He also obtained his best results when first cleansing the colon of all putrefactive material. In the same year, Lieutenant H. V. Hughens, United States Medical Corps, improved on Dr. Norman's apparatus.[4] Both Norman and Hughens implanted acidophilus rectally after emptying the colon. Although no information is currently available on the source of the culture used by either practitioner, they did report excellent results. Unfortunately, with the advent of antibiotics, which doctors quickly adopted as *the* therapy of choice for all bacterial infections, Norman and Hughens's work was eclipsed.

Today, of course, we know all too well the impact of antibiotics on the acidophilus colon flora. Both bad and good bacteria are killed at once. For the short-term relief we have gained, we now suffer long-term damage to our health and immunity. Blinded by the power of antibiotics, science overlooked the knowledge it had gained about the importance of maintaining the healthy acidophilus colon flora itself.

David Webster—Into the Twenty-first Century

I was led to this work through an unexpected event in my normally healthy and busy life. I awoke one morning in excruciating pain, unable to get out of bed. Several visits to doctors were inconclusive; they were unable to diagnose or alleviate my pain. After one visit with Dr. Gibson, a chiropractor, who gave me a colonic, I walked out of her office pain-free and have never had the problem recur in the past 24 years. She said my condition was a sciatic nerve attack due to toxicity and impaction in my colon. She explained that the sciatic nerve, the largest nerve in the body, can become inflamed due to accumulation of toxins in the unhealthy colon. My interest was captured.

The next day I spoke with the owner of my favorite local health food store, who, in his eighties, was in excellent health. I told him of my experience and that while researching the colon I had read about the importance of replacing my natural acidophilus flora. I asked him to recommend a strain of acidophilus that would be effective. He explained the necessity of using human-strain acidophilus and of implanting it rectally. Since I was so interested, he gave me a rare, out-of-print manuscript to read. This was my introduction to the writings of Dr. Empringham, which also inspired me to apply his research and eventually led to the writing of this book.

After applying Empringham's information with good results, I extended my research to several large medical libraries and uncovered a wealth of studies and information. I quickly realized the importance of this missing link in our current medical knowledge. Over more than 20 years I have gathered information and combined various areas of medical, nutritional, and microbiological research with clinical experience to form a complete picture of colon health. Both ancient medical wisdom and modern scientific research have inspired me. The role of colon flora in overall health is indeed great. You, too, can attain and maintain your colon health. From my research, then, I have added the following ten important tenets to those of Metchnikoff and Empringham:

1. By definition, the healthy adult colon is at a slightly acid pH of 5.6 to 6.9 and houses bacteria, the majority of which are the protective acidophilus.
2. The acidophilus colon flora supports our health and immune system. The flora's slightly acid secretions act as a protective barrier to prevent harmful microbes, yeast, parasites, and other pathogens from taking hold.
3. Almost everyone today has a deficient or depleted colon flora due to our unhealthy modern lifestyle.

4. It is necessary to follow specific steps to reestablish a deficient or depleted colon flora with lasting results.
5. The most important factor in reestablishing colon health is to create a slightly acid environment favorable for acidophilus growth and proliferation.
6. Taking acidophilus orally will not change the alkaline, pathogenic colon flora or reestablish the protective flora we need.
7. Water colonics, water enemas, or colon cleanse products do not reestablish a healthy colon because they leave the colon in an alkaline condition.
8. Edible-grade, sweet whole whey, used regularly, is the overall best single food to benefit the acidophilus flora because:
   a. It provides lactose and other nutrients required by the acidophilus flora for their growth.
   b. It works as an antiseptic to cleanse and reacidify the colon gently.
9. It is possible to restore a deficient colon flora by supplying it with human-grade, sweet, whole whey orally in the daily diet.
10. A severely depleted colon flora requires cleansing and reacidification of the colon followed by:
    a. A rectal implant of a good-quality, human-grade acidophilus culture.
    b. Proper maintenance by using sweet whole whey orally, to ensure proliferation and growth of the implanted flora.

All these important principles will be explained clearly as we proceed in our understanding of acidophilus and colon health.

Questions and Answers

Q. *Why hasn't the research about acidophilus and colon health been more well known?*

A. I am constantly asked this question. In the 1930s there was quite a lot of research published about acidophilus. In fact, while some medical professionals performed colon cleansing to clear focal infections, others used replacement therapy after cleansing to restore health. As we will explore further, though, the advent of antibiotics in the 1940s eclipsed all other lines of research. In 1980, when I first published this book in pamphlet form, I brought many of the old studies to light again.

Q. *How do I know if I can just drink whey mixed with water to replenish my colon flora or if I need to implant the acidophilus and whey rectally?*

A. Most people still have some colonics of acidophilus alive in their colon that can be restored and encouraged to multiply by providing them with nutrients. This can be accomplished by drinking whey on a daily basis. The stool will usually improve and reflect a healthy colon flora within eight weeks. If no changes are seen in this time, it is likely that the colon is too deficient in acidophilus, contains too much toxic material, or is too weak to sustain an acidophilus colony in an alkaline pH. In this case, a whey enema followed by a rectal implant of acidophilus is indicated. This is described in more detail later on.

Q. *Can you give an example of a pathogen?*

A. The same toxic bacteria that cause degenerative conditions decompose dead bodies. Many people harbor these pathogenic bacteria in their colons, which slowly break down the immune system.

2

IN THE BEGINNING

■

From our first taste of mother's milk to our last breath, the normal colon flora is absolutely essential for our survival throughout life. At birth, breast milk provides an infant the foundation necessary to form a strong immune system. In the first few days of life, breast milk is the link that extends a mother's immunity to her infant. The antibodies in mother's milk offer the infant protection against the microorganisms capable of producing disease.

In addition to antibodies, we receive an initial culture of beneficial bacteria from our mother's breast milk. Mother's milk contains *Bifidobacterium bifidum* and specific growth factors for *B. bifidum* along with important immunoglobulins. *B. bifidum* flourishes on the high level of lactose and other nutrients contained in breast milk.[1] These bacteria all help to establish the basis for a strong immune system in the new infant. Usually within the first few days of breastfeeding, the colon of a breastfed infant contains about 99 percent *Bifidobacterium bifidum.* Other bacteria, such as enterococci and coliform, constitute about 1 percent of the colon population.[2,3]

This high percentage of *B. bifidum* in an infant's colon

is referred to as a "simplified flora." Because the simplified flora acts as a vital barrier to infections, breastfed babies are found to have greater resistance to infection and better health than formula-fed infants.[4,5] Bottle-fed infants do not do as well. Although the colon flora of bottle-fed infants contains many species of bacteria, there are fewer beneficial bacteria and little, if any, B. bifidum.[6] Formula-fed infants are also more susceptible to irritability, colic, and infection. In response, doctors commonly prescribe antibiotics for such infants, resulting in a further weakened immune system, which can adversely affect their health for life.[7]

During breastfeeding, infants are less likely to experience allergies or asthma than bottle-fed babies.[8] When infants drink formulas made from cow's milk during their first year of life, an allergic response can also be triggered that will affect their digestive tract, lungs, blood, and skin. Nearly 25 percent of infants who are allergic to cow's milk are also allergic to soy, which is commonly used as an alternative in infant formulas. When breastfeeding is not possible, some experts advise mothers to feed their babies hydrolyzed whey formula to avoid the allergic response to milk or soy proteins.[9] Goat's milk is another option worth considering. Of course, in your search for a formula most appropriate for your infant, a compassionate and knowledgeable physician can be of great help—so don't fail to consult with a physician you trust.

There are many excellent reasons for women to breastfeed. For example, a woman who nurses her baby for longer than 4 to 6 months is 49 percent less likely to develop breast cancer throughout her lifetime.[10] Breastfeeding fosters a nurturing bond between mother and infant. In addition, breastfeeding provides the nutrient and bacterial foundation for a strong immune system. Of interest here as well is a recent study that showed breastfed infants have fewer ear infections (otitis media) than bottle-fed infants. In fact, the risk of ear infection decreased significantly in 289 children for up to 4 months after breastfeeding was discontinued.[11] When breastfeeding implants the protective flora in the infant's colon at birth, and he or she maintains it throughout life, it can make a sizable contribution to sustained health.

Due to the acid-loving and acid-secreting *B. bifidum*, the colon of a breastfed infant is slightly acid. And well it is for the infant, for a slightly acidic colon prevents the growth of harmful pathogenic bacteria, which can thrive only in an alkaline environment. In addition to these mild acids, other factors in acidophilus secretions have been found to exert antagonistic actions on the growth of specific pathogenic bacteria.[12]

As an infant grows and begins to eat food, more types of bacteria appear in the colon. *Lactobacillus acidophilus* and other beneficial strains appear, along with some pathogenic bacteria carried on food. Then the flora naturally changes from the simplified colon flora of a breastfed infant to a more complex or mixed flora. In an adult, a healthy colon flora consists of about 80 to 85 percent protective acidophilus flora with 15 to 20 percent of other types of bacteria. This balance can be maintained through proper diet and lifestyle to ensure the slightly acid pH essential for a healthy colon and a strong immune system throughout life. Many factors can and will upset this delicate balance, allowing harmful bacteria to gain the upper hand. Formula-fed infants, for example, start off with an unbalanced colon flora. Fortunately it is possible to transform an unhealthy colon flora and restore the healthy balance of protective bacteria in the colon at any time in life.

Questions and Answers

Q. *Does the acidophilus flora become depleted with age?*

A. Age is not a factor as much as industrialization, which has changed the food we eat dramatically. Metchnikoff studied country people who maintained their traditional diet and lifestyle. He found they used yogurt containing whey, which they made for centuries. These people maintained their original beneficial colon flora throughout life.

3

COLON FLORA: OUR PROTECTIVE SHIELD

■

There is a direct correlation between the colon flora and a person's health. Studies in earlier decades, especially the 1930s and 1940s, suggest that a normal acidophilus flora predominant in the colon helps prevent many degenerative conditions such as arthritis, neuritis, bursitis, colitis, and diverticulitis.[1,2,3,4,5] Unfortunately, modern medicine treats disease symptomatically because the foundation of knowledge we have regarding the root cause of inflammatory and degenerative conditions has been discarded. Quite simply, pathogenic colon bacteria excrete molecular toxic waste into the human system, which can cause inflammations and degenerative disease. On the other hand, beneficial colon bacteria function as part of the immune system and secrete nutrients assimilated into the human system.

The word "acidophilus" means "acid-loving." "Flora" means "flower" and refers here to the microenvironment of bacteria in the colon. All bacteria are minute living organisms with specific growth and nutrient requirements. For their part, human acidophilus bacteria are very delicate organisms. They are also anaerobic, which means they can

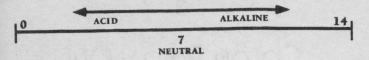

Figure 1. Basic pH Chart

live only in oxygen-free environments. As we have seen, acidophilus can live only in a specific range of a slightly acid pH.

pH and Health

The chemical term "pH" refers to the relative acidity or alkalinity of a substance or environment. This measure is determined by the concentration of hydrogen ions in a solution. The higher the concentration of ions, the more active and "acidic" the solution. Solutions with a lower concentration of hydrogen ions are "alkaline." pH is measured in a range of 0 to 14. A pH value of 7 is neutral and is called a "buffer," as it is neither acid nor alkaline. Anything below 7 is acid and above 7 is alkaline. The increase in pH is geometrical, which means that a pH of 6 is ten times more acid than a pH of 7. A pH of 5 is one hundred times more acid than a pH of 7.

At the cellular level, this activity of hydrogen ions in a solution, measured as pH, forms the basis of metabolic activity in our bodies. Every aspect of the body functions within a very specific pH range. Outside of that range disease, malfunction, and even sudden death can result.

In health, the pH of the blood, saliva, extracellular fluid, and lower small intestine should be alkaline. The pH of the stomach, urine, colon, and skin should be acid.

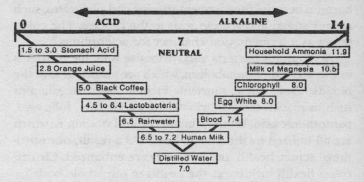

Figure 2. Substance pH Chart[6,7,8]

Extracellular fluid bathes all the cells in our body. In health, this fluid is slightly alkaline, in the range of 7.35 to 7.45. Life can exist when the extracellular fluid is in the pH range of 6.8 to 7.8, but these are the outer limits.

Blood pH should be in the range of 7.35 to 7.45. If it becomes just a little too acid, life-threatening conditions will follow. If the blood becomes too alkaline, other lesser problems can arise.

The skin acts as an antiseptic protective mantle because of its slightly acid pH provided by nature. This helps prevent inflammatory bacteria on our skin from causing infection. When the skin is broken, however, infection can follow. The reason is simple: Bacteria that were held in check by the acid pH of the skin can now migrate fully into the alkaline bloodstream, where they begin to multiply.

Likewise, the interior lining of the colon must be in a slightly acid, antiseptic condition to prevent internal infections from developing in the colon and from penetrating into the body. Acidophilus create the very pH they themselves require. Acidophilus are known as a fermentative bacteria because they ferment specific carbohydrates, such as milk sugar, and secrete acids in the process. The colon serves as a fermentation chamber for acidophilus.[9]

Acidophilus bacteria also synthesize valuable nutrients in the process of metabolism, which are absorbed into the bloodstream. These nutrients include essential vitamins such as niacin, thiamin, riboflavin, pyridoxine, folic acid, pantothenic acid, biotin, vitamin B_{12}, and vitamin K, which are all utilized by the human host.[10] As a result, our nutritional status, health and immunity are enhanced. Clearly, colon health influences the health of our whole body.

The prevalence of an alkaline colon has led many health professionals and laypersons to the misconception that the "normal" colon pH is slightly alkaline. *Taber's Medical Dictionary*, for example, states that for an infant, the normal stool pH is usually acid, while for adults, the normal stool pH is neutral or alkaline.[11] Although this may be very common, it is not normal. Why does this contradiction exist? An unfortunate fact of current medical science is how it defines a "normal" lab test reading. An average is calculated from all readings over a recent period. This average is then considered to indicate a "normal" reading. Unfortunately, with the decline of health in the general population in the past 50 years, "normal" readings only reflect a continually lowering standard of health.

Certainly, this situation needs to be remedied. "Normal" readings should be based on results of lab tests from healthy individuals to accurately reflect levels of optimal health and functioning. When the adult colon is maintained at a slightly acidic pH of 5.6 to 6.9, fostering a predominantly acidophilus flora, this vital living part of our immune system is working as nature intended.

Digestive System and Immune Function

The digestive system functions in a unique way as part of the body's immune defense system. In fact, it protects us from invasion by harmful bacteria and other pathogens due to the great variation of pH values between the stomach, small intestine, and colon.

First, the stomach's highly acid secretions kill most foreign microbes such as bacteria. The stomach contains very strong acids to prevent food from spoiling in the body, to digest components of our food, and to kill harmful bacteria and other pathogens. Stomach pH ranges from 1.5 (very acidic) to 3.0 (medium acidic), depending on the stomach's stage of digestion or rest.[12] When too little acid is produced in the stomach, digestion is hampered. When acid production is high, on the other hand, the lining of the stomach will be eaten away over time, resulting in ulcers.

After leaving the stomach, food enters the small intestine, which has an alkaline pH essential for further breakdown and assimilation of nutrients. Scientific data point out that, in a healthy state, the small intestine is sterile.[13] It is not normally inhabited by a bacterial population and any bacteria present in the small intestine are transient—just passing through.

The small intestine empties into the ascending colon at the ileocecal valve. The cecum is a tough, thick pouch that lies beneath the ascending colon, to which the appendix is attached. It provides an important function for colon health. When the small intestine empties into the ascending colon, the cecum contracts, mixing the food and pushing it along. In a healthy colon, fecal matter is

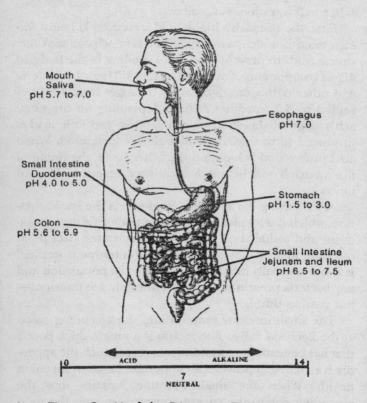

Mouth
Saliva
pH 5.7 to 7.0

Esophagus
pH 7.0

Small Intestine
Duodenum
pH 4.0 to 5.0

Stomach
pH 1.5 to 3.0

Colon
pH 5.6 to 6.9

Small Intestine
Jejunem and Ileum
pH 6.5 to 7.5

0   ACID   ALKALINE   14

7
NEUTRAL

Figure 3. pH of the Digestive Tract in Health

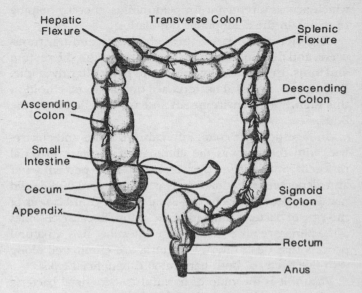

Figure 4. Colon Anatomy

pushed along by contractions of the muscular colon wall called peristalsis. When there are no acidophilus present, the cecum becomes weak and sluggish. Fecal or food residues can remain in the cecum or ascending colon and may not be pushed along properly for elimination. In this small pouch, harmful bacteria and toxins can accumulate. Far Eastern nomadic tribes used this mechanism quite well. They stored their milk, for example, in leather containers with a small pouch at the bottom. The small pouch retained milk cultures to acidify any fresh milk added to the container. Metchnikoff and others state that the cecum is intended to function in a similar manner.[14] *B. bifidum* implanted in a breastfed baby multiplies in the cecum, which acts as a reservoir for acidophilus, thereby helping to maintain the acidophilus population.

Digested food passes through the ascending, transverse, and descending colon and out through the rectum and anus. In the healthy colon, the pH is slightly acidic. Pathogenic, harmful bacteria are unable to take hold in this slightly acid environment and are expelled from the body.

In digestion, the colon will reabsorb fluids and electrolytes into the body as the elimination of waste material proceeds. Studies show that feces contain 75 percent water and 25 percent solid matter. Nearly 30 percent of the solid matter in feces is bacteria—usually a good indication of the type of bacteria inhabiting the colon. Because colonies of bacteria are alive in the large intestine, it is a natural process that dead "waste" bacteria are eliminated along with live bacteria, both harmful and beneficial types.

Again, it is the ratio of harmful to beneficial bacteria that is most important for health. When the colon is slightly acid, with a predominance of acidophilus, the excess pathogenic bacteria are eliminated and balance is maintained within the colon chamber. Indicators of a healthy colon flora are a soft but well-formed stool, with amber color and little or no odor, and that floats in water most of the time. When the stools are dry, dark brown, too solidly formed, or too loose, and especially if there is a putrid odor, these are clear indicators of a putrefactive, alkaline-producing colon flora. Chronic constipation, diarrhea, and irritable bowel syndrome are often eliminated when the colon is restored and maintained at a slightly acid pH.

When undigested food is present in the bowel movement, it shows there is poor digestion. The colon does not break down foods and is not meant to deal with undigested food particles. When poorly digested food reaches the

TABLE 1.
A Healthy and Unhealthy Stool

	Healthy Stool	Unhealthy Stool
pH	Slightly acidic	Alkaline
Predominant populations	Lactobacteria	Pathogens
Odor	None	Foul or strong odor
Color	Medium brown	Chalky, black, dark brown, gray
Form	Well formed	Loose, stringy, hard balls
Buoyancy	Floats most of the time	Seldom or never floats
Pattern	Consistent	Inconsistent
Regularity	1 to 2 times a day	Less than once a day or more than 3 times a day
Other factors	No mucus, blood, or undigested food particles	Presence of blood, mucus, or undigested food particles

colon on a regular basis, it can contribute to the formation of an alkaline colon. Digestive enzymes can often assist proper digestion. In this regard, plant enzymes are usually very effective. You can observe the result by checking your stools. If your normal digestive supplement or the enzymes from plants you eat do not help to form healthy stools, you may need to consult your doctor and possibly have tests to determine whether you have stomach acids sufficient for digestion.

Homeostasis, Health, and Immunity

Homeostasis refers to regulatory processes that maintain the body's internal constancy. In fact, homeostasis is a term that describes how the body survives. No matter what our lifestyle or health habits, the body strives to maintain all functions necessary for life. As inner and outer conditions change, the body adjusts or compensates to sustain health. In this light, homeostasis is a compensatory function. This is why, even under less-than-optimal conditions, the body will function and maintain some outer semblance of health.

People with poor digestion or even those suffering from alcoholism often appear healthy for many years. Here, homeostasis is at work. Nonetheless, homeostasis does operate within certain limits. In effect, the body will adjust but only so far. The blood, which will not tolerate even minute changes in pH without dramatic effects, including possible death, is another story entirely. Other tissues or organs will tolerate greater changes in pH for varying amounts of time. A change in the urine's pH can quickly result in a urinary tract infection, while a change in the stomach's pH takes much longer to result in noticeable health problems.

Unlike most areas of the body, the colon does not possess sensory nerves. Without such nerves, there is no way for us to feel the onset or progression of problems in the area. A colon condition must reach a severe state before we feel or notice it. In this light, an alkaline colon pH acts as a quiet, continuous, and insidious contributor to disease. It takes many years, in fact, for an alkaline colon to lead to health problems, seemingly much more common today than in the past. The rise in the incidence of inflammatory

TABLE 2.
A Healthy Adult Colon

A Healthy Adult Colon	
pH	Slightly acid in the range of 5.6 to 6.9.
Predominant bacteria	Fermentative bacteria such as *L. acidophilus* and *B. bifidum*.
Bacterial secretions	Slightly acid by-products as a result of their action on foods. Produces nutrients, such as B vitamins and vitamin K, absorbed into the bloodstream.
Immune function	Acidophilus flora serves as a protective barrier to prevent harmful microbes, parasites, pathogens, and their toxic by-products from taking hold in the body.
Colon function	Acts as an absorption chamber. Water, electrolytes and nutrients are absorbed into the body.
Cecum function	Acts as a reservoir for a starter culture of acidophilus bacteria.
Stool	No odor and no gas production.

and leaky gut conditions, which are felt or noticed only in their advanced stages, is just another indication of how long it takes for us to respond therapeutically. For this reason, it is wise to maintain the colon in a slightly acid state and promote the proliferation of an acidophilus flora as a preventive health measure.

The role of the digestive system in immunity is to provide a strong line of defense against invasion by bacteria and other pathogens. Without an acidophilus colon flora, this part of our immune system is at best nonfunctioning

TABLE 3.
An Unhealthy Adult Colon

An Unhealthy Adult Colon	
pH	Alkaline in pH.
Predominant bacteria	Putrefactive, pathogenic bacteria.
Bacterial secretions	Form toxic by-products that are absorbed into the bloodstream and are damaging to health.
Immune function	No immune function due to lack of protective flora. Harmful to immune system due to toxic by-products.
Colon function	Impairment of absorption of water and nutrients.
Cecum function	Becomes a reservoir of pathogenic bacteria.
Stool	Bad odor and gas production.

and at worse a breeding chamber for harmful bacteria and other opportunists.

Questions and Answers

Q. *How does colon pH affect the rest of the body?*

A. The pH of the entire system is based in the colon flora. You can read Chapter 6, "Keys to Health: Colon and Liver," to understand this better. In the same chapter, Figure 5 shows the pathway for this influence. Metabolic by-products from the colon flora enter the bloodstream from the colon. These by-products affect the chemical content of pH of the blood, which, in turn, affects the rest of the body.

4

DEFENSE BETRAYED: PROTECTIVE SHIELD DESTROYED

■

Numerous factors are involved in destroying the beneficial acidophilus bacteria, including medication, drugs, poor diet, and stress, which then affects the condition and population of the more general colon flora.[1]

Over the past hundred years, with the growth of industrialization and the rise in population, our immune system has suffered and, in many cases, broken down completely. I include in this degenerative process a concomitant breakdown of the protective shield of our natural colon flora. This breakdown has allowed the invasion of harmful microorganisms and contributed to the formation of many chronic and other serious diseases.

You might want to ask yourself a very obvious question at this point: "How many of my physical and emotional problems began after taking modern medications, after eating foods that carry pesticides, after living in a smogbound city?" and so on. I'm sure that the answer will not surprise you. In terms of the acidophilus colon flora, antibiotics in particular have well-known adverse effects. In the 1940s, antibiotics, the new "magic bullets" against disease, became the focus of modern medicine. While

TABLE 4.
Factors That Harm the Acidophilus Flora

Factors that harm our acidophilus flora:

- Pharmaceutical drugs including
  - Antibiotics
  - Nonprescription drugs
  - Steroids
  - Birth control pills
- Street or "recreational" drugs
- Alcohol
- Pesticides
- Pollution
- Laxatives
- Poor nutrition and diet
  - Excess fat or protein consumption
  - Food additives and preservatives
- High stress
- Trauma
- Exposure to microorganisms in food and in the environment
- Constitution and health of the individual

health professionals as far back as 1950 recognized that antibiotics destroy the acidophilus colon flora, no effective steps were taken then, or are usually taken now, to replenish this natural flora after a patient completes a course of antibiotic therapy.

Used correctly, of course, antibiotics do save lives. On the other hand, antibiotics kill bacteria without differentiating between types, whether harmful or beneficial. With antibiotics, the acidophilus flora is no longer predominant and the colon pH is no longer slightly acid—as it should be. As it turns alkaline, the colon becomes perfect terrain for the growth of pathogenic microorganisms. These pathogens can then take hold and become a source of many toxic, metabolic by-products that directly or indirectly harm the human immune system.

Antibiotic Overuse

Nature intended microorganisms and humans to coexist. Both life and death are dependent on bacterial support. Many microorganisms are harmless. Some, such as the colon acidophilus, play a specific role in the human life cycle. Others damage our system and a few microorganisms are even lethal.

In this regard, "antibiosis," the process whereby one microorganism destroys the life of another in order to sustain its own life,[2] is important to understand as a precurser to antibiotics, which were finally discovered in the 1920s by Sir Alexander Fleming, a Scottish bacteriologist and physician. He observed that an agar plate inoculated with *Staphylococcus aureus* had become contaminated with a mold colony. He also noted a clear zone surrounding the mold colony, indicating inhibition of bacterial growth.

Fleming then identified the mold and studied its anti-bacterial activities.[3] During World War II, as penicillin use proliferated, it saved thousands of lives from the scourge of bacteria-related infections.

Since then, bacteria have become increasingly resistant to antibiotics as Stuart Levy, M.D., eloquently described in his book *The Antibiotic Paradox*. Recognized internationally as an expert in antibiotic use and bacterial resistance to antibiotics, Dr. Levy is a professor of medicine, molecular biology, and microbiology at Tufts University School of Medicine.

According to Levy, microorganisms adjust and evolve at very fast rates. In fact, they have adjusted to every imaginable chemical produced by man, and now can survive many chemicals they could not before. Researchers are challenged to keep our drug arsenals current with the fast mutation rate of microbes, multidrug regimens included. In this regard, Dr. Levy was the first to document the transfer of multidrug resistance between animals and humans. He also discovered the mechanism for resistance to the well-known antibiotic oxytetracycline.

Antibiotic resistance can be triggered in several ways. Our use and abuse of mercury in dentistry provides a pertinent example. In the early 1800s, mercury was first used for amalgam dental fillings. From that time till recently medical authorities believed that mercury would not pass from the tooth to the body. In the 1980s, however, a research team observed that mercury caused bacteria to become antibiotic resistant. In 1993, a study of 640 individuals at the University of Georgia, Athens, indicated that amalgam tooth fillings were a contributing factor to antibiotic resistance. Contact with mercury can also cause genetic changes in human oral and intestinal bacteria.

Those bacteria that are not destroyed by mercury acquire genetic resistance to the toxicity of mercury.[4]

Dr. Levy goes on to describe the ability of bacteria to convey drug-resistant information among each other and even to dissimilar bacterial species. Penicillin, for example, is currently ineffective against many strains of gonorrhea found worldwide. In Africa, 50 percent of the bacteria that cause cholera are resistant to tetracycline.[5] New strains of tuberculosis are now resistant to most, if not all, available antibiotics. Difficult-to-treat and lingering ear infections are also becoming more common in children. In response, children are sometimes kept on antibiotics for years without positive results.

Without changing our minds about how to treat bacterial infections and disease, this situation can only get worse. Because microorganisms constantly readjust to their environment and become progressively resistant even to multidrug regimens, physicians have responded almost by rote: prescribing *stronger* doses of antibiotics over time. The use of increased dosages, along with the widespread frequency of such prescriptions, has seriously damaged our protective shield, the beneficial colon flora, provided by nature to humans at birth. Our entire immune system suffers defeat as we become deficient in our normal levels of beneficial flora.

Misuse of antibiotics and other drugs is analogous to tending a garden by using a shovel to turn the soil to get rid of the weeds but forgetting thereafter to fertilize the soil and to plant seeds. In this scenario, planting ground cover, whether flowers or crops, is neglected and the weeds return, growing more wildly and vigorously than ever before.

Nature intended the friendly acidophilus flora to be our front-line defense against microbial invaders. Without

this protection, we suffer. For every force, there is a coun-
terforce. It seems that the microcosm of invisible microorganisms is taking over the earth. We have won the battle
and are rapidly losing the war!

Environmental Factors

Commercial and processed foods also contribute to
damaging the colon flora. The early 1900s brought dramatic changes in the food-processing industry. Liquid and
hydrogenated vegetable oils were manufactured by a process requiring the use of harsh chemicals and high temperatures. Convenience foods, devitalized by processing
methods to extend shelf life, have become a common way
of eating. Pesticides, which are an outgrowth of the coal
tar and nerve gas industries, are pervasive in the food
chain. Pesticides are present in all our commercially grown
crops and in animal foods because the animals are eating
chemically sprayed foods and grasses.

Many pesticides mimic estrogen in the body, which
disrupts normal endocrine (hormonal) function, causes
excess estrogenic activity, and leads to many diseases
including cancer. Scientists have found endocrine-dis-
rupting contaminants to be present in living tissue at con-
centrations millions of times higher than the natural
hormones.

Besides being well known as hormone disrupters, pesticides and herbicides also suppress the immune system and
cause other serious health problems. These are long-term
effects that can take years or even decades to manifest and
are complicated by continual exposure to a multitude of
chemicals in the course of our daily lives. No specific studies have ever been done on the effect of pesticides as they

accumulate in the human body or on the interaction of the many different kinds of pesticides within the human body over long periods of time.

Nonetheless, these dietary and chemical factors that were introduced into our lives during the early 1900s, combined with environmental factors and medical drugs, have damaged our natural colon flora along with our overall immune function and health.

The colon must be reacidified to restore health. If it is not, a person can relapse and his or her overall health will suffer in the long run. Following appropriate use of antibiotics, for example, a postantibiotic therapy is needed to *replenish* the normal colon flora. Historically, no such therapy has been applied. The current recommendations that people "eat yogurt" or "take acidophilus supplements" are based on faulty information and will not replenish the damaged colon flora. In Chapter 9, we will see the reasons why. First, however, we will explore just how an unhealthy colon can adversely affect our well-being.

Questions and Answers

Q. *You've described the effects of chemicals and drugs. Will natural products such as herbs or nutritional products destroy the beneficial bacteria as well?*

A. Some natural substances can damage the flora. Herbs such as goldenseal and raw garlic act as natural antibiotics that can harm beneficial as well as pathogenic bacteria. Raw garlic irritates the digestive tract and can be harmful to the acidophilus colon flora. The health benefits of garlic can be gained by using a liquid preparation of specially aged garlic that also actually benefits the colon flora.

Herbal, coffee, or wheatgrass enemas also leave the colon in an alkaline condition, vulnerable to invasion by pathogenic bacteria. If herbal or coffee enemas are recommended by your health practitioner, show him or her this information.

Q. *What is colloidal silver and how does it affect the colon flora?*

A. Colloidal silver is being used as a natural alternative to antibiotics because it is found to be antibacterial and even antiviral. Silver is a toxic mineral, which is, however, an essential mineral required by the body in minute amounts. Colloidal silver is a special preparation where silver particles are suspended in liquid. Colloids often have an electrical charge that interacts with the body at a cellular level.

While some good results are being obtained with its clinical use, colloidal silver appears to negatively affect the acidophilus colon flora. I have had several clients return for another implant due to taking colloidal silver. They all felt fine and much improved after reestablishing their healthy colon flora. As soon as they took colloidal silver, their colon problems returned. Once they reacidified their colon and reestablished the acidophilus flora, their health improved again.

Q. *I have prostate problems. Is the colon flora a possible cause?*

A. The prostate sits in direct contact with the colon. If the colon is alkaline and creating molecular toxic by-products, these can be absorbed directly through the tissues into the prostate. The best way to prevent prostate problems is to eliminate the cause at its source.

5

THE TOXIC COLON

■

When antibiotic or other drug therapy destroys the resident acidophilus, the colon becomes susceptible to the next line of aggressors: pathogens, yeasts, parasites, and viruses.

This happens because only harmful bacteria will proliferate in the alkaline colon. Harmful bacteria in turn continue to create an alkaline, putrefactive environment instead of the normal acidic, fermentative balance. Pathogenic bacteria take over the entire colon and secrete poisons as a result of their metabolic activity. These toxins include skatole, hydrogen sulfide, histamine, tyramine, indole, phenol, cadaverin, and many others.[1] They are transported from the colon through the mesenteric vein, into the portal vein, and into the liver (for visual clarification here, you may wish to refer to Figure 5, Chapter 6). Many of these toxins, however, then spill over into the bloodstream, where they circulate and contribute to depression of the central nervous system and other effects.[2]

The liver's filtration capacity to detoxify impurities becomes challenged after many years of pollution. When the liver becomes overwhelmed and clogged, the bloodstream, kidneys, and bladder are then affected. The result is common: inefficient elimination and a weakened immune system.

In the normal, healthy colon, yeasts are typically present at a ratio of 1 yeast per 1,000 acidophilus. Present in this ratio, yeasts do no harm. When the colon flora becomes abnormal, however, this ratio can reverse to as few as 1 acidophilus per 1,000 yeast, with ill health the result as noted.[3] Over 150 yeast species have been isolated in different infections.[4] The most common yeast culprit, responsible for many clinical syndromes, is *Candida albicans.* When the normal colon flora is destroyed by antibiotics, birth control pills, or medications such as steroids, *Candida* can overgrow on the mucosal surfaces of the mouth, colon, and vagina. Although the Centers for Disease Control (CDC) do not recognize *Candida* as a communicable disease, we know differently. Authorities who describe *Candida* as being transmitted by sexual contact, by the hands of medical attendants, and from the mother's birth canal to the infant are precise on this point.[5]

Candida

You may recognize some of the following symptoms of *Candida albicans:* fungus under the nails, in the mouth, or in the vagina; headaches; indigestion; colon malfunction; bloating; menstrual cramps; allergies; food sensitivities; chronic fatigue syndrome; and others.

Candida is an opportunistic organism, classified as a yeast/fungus. With the destruction of acidophilus, the colon pH changes from acid to alkaline, which sets up perfect conditions for overgrowth of *Candida* and other pathogens. When the immune system is weakened by any cause, an opportunity arises for *Candida* to rapidly multiply, creating and releasing highly toxic substances into the system. *Candida* can penetrate the mucosal lining of the colon, allowing minute particles of undigested protein to enter the system and trigger allergic reactions. As long as *Candida* predominates in the colon, symptoms will continue to recur in other parts of the body.

It is possible to control *Candida* with known antifungal remedies. Following use of these antifungal remedies, immediate replacement of acidophilus to restore their acid production in the colon (and the vagina in women) is essential to prevent a relapse. Unfortunately doctors routinely misdiagnose people as having yeast infections such as *Candida* without laboratory confirmation. It is important to determine by laboratory analysis whether yeasts are present at harmful levels in the system and if *Candida* is actually the culprit.

Scientists culturing *Candida* in the laboratory have found a relationship between *Candida* growth, acidophilus growth, and the colon environment. When laboratory culture media are vitamin-deficient, *Candida* thrives. Acidophilus, on the other hand, require specific nutrients, including riboflavin, niacin, pantothenate, pyridoxine, and others. Thus, in the human body, a nutritious diet will support an existing healthy flora. In laboratory conditions, the population of yeasts is reduced when the pH is slightly acid, between 5.3 and 5.8. In the human body, this acid pH is maintained as a result of the lactic and other acids secreted by the acidophilus colon flora. Thus, when acidophilus predominate in the colon and a person's nutrition is adequate, *Candida* will not be able to take hold in the system. There can only be disease where there is a medium!

Parasites

Candida is just one example of what can happen when the colon flora is thrown off balance. In a toxic colon, many other harmful bacteria and microorganisms, including parasites, can thrive and multiply.

By definition, parasites require the support of a host to sustain them. They depend on predigested food from their host. Parasitic infection can be chronic or acute, with symptoms ranging from none to severe. Within this range of symptoms, people may complain of constipation, diarrhea, irritable bowel syndrome, fatigue, edema, low back pain, sciatica, frequent nasal draining, and even bad gas. Gas and bloating may be constant and increase after meals. Other signs may include hunger even after eating a meal, craving sugar, weight loss or gain, and iron-deficiency anemia.

Although it is not always accurate, the most effective method of diagnosis is through stool analysis. Be careful, though. Because current stool analysis is not sophisticated enough to detect parasites under all conditions, you may need to repeat the analysis several times.

A person you may know or meet may also be a carrier without having an obvious infection. Parasites can survive in low numbers and then multiply and spread rapidly when the host's resistance drops due to high stress, nutrient deficiency, trauma, or sudden or chronic illness. Parasites that used to be considered harmless, such as *Cryptosporidium,* for example, cause serious illnesses and even death in people chronically ill with viral or autoimmune diseases.

In the past few years, parasites have been causing more problems than ever before. Even as parasitic infections are on the rise, many people and even health practitioners still consider parasites to be exclusively a Third World problem. This is not the case! Along with the increase in world travel, the distribution of parasites has become widespread. After traveling to places such as India, Bali, or South America, people sometimes become quite ill within a four-week period—the usual incubation time for many parasitic eggs to hatch.

Parasites infect people through many different pathways. Transmission can take place directly through polluted water, food, and soil, or from contact with infected animals or insects. Parasites are found throughout the world. Although tropical temperatures and humidity favor parasites, besides their abundance in Third World countries, they also commonly occur in North America, Canada, Alaska, and Russia. Of course, low temperatures usually prevent eggs and larvae from developing. On the other hand, if you are infected, your bodily moisture and warmth—the perfect medium for parasites—will activate them.

Nor are advanced farming and harvesting techniques parasite clean. Some parasites can even be found on the best-quality produce. In this regard, it's best to be cautious when visiting open salad bars and restaurants offering freshly squeezed vegetable juices. Because we cannot see contaminants on our food without using a microscope does not mean they are absent. Always wash, scrape, and peel raw foods before eating them. This sounds like common sense, but it is amazing how many people still eat food directly from the produce section of the supermarket or health food store without first washing it well. In addition, while the label "organically grown" is meaningful to the consumer, in terms of how the food was farmed, it is meaningless to the parasite, who does not distinguish between organic and chemically grown foods.

Remember as well that most parasites are destroyed at

cooking temperatures. Thus, despite the growing popularity of sushi in the American diet, think before you take that bite of raw fish: You are gambling with your health! A fisherman opening a freshly caught fish to find a belly full of worms is a sight you will never forget. Worm larvae may exist even in the best-quality fish. There is no way to confirm their presence without a microscope, so why take chances? Cook most of your foods, especially your fish!

If laboratory analysis detects a parasite infection in you, either chemical or natural remedies can be prescribed. For severe parasitic infections chemical treatment is much more effective. The infected individual must comply fully with the course of treatment, however, and follow particular hygiene practices. The house, toilets, bedding, and yard should be kept as clean as possible. Hands must be clean for food preparation and eating. Children should also be taught to wash their hands after going to the bathroom, petting animals, or playing outside.

People who suffer from parasitic infections usually find only temporary relief from current therapies. In many cases, while treatment is successful initially, relapse occurs soon after. The reason is simple: Once the parasites are killed off, eggs may remain. The colon must immediately be restored to its acid pH and acidophilus flora to prevent relapse as well. When parasites are correctly identified and destroyed, debris from the breakdown of the dead parasites will reach the colon. If the colon is already in an unhealthy state, these end products will cause further problems. If the infection is massive, even the normal colon flora can be overwhelmed.

After the infection has been correctly diagnosed and the parasites have been destroyed, the colon should be cleansed promptly to remove any dead parasites and putrefaction. Then the natural flora must be immediately restored, so the colon can regain its natural slightly acid state and resume normal functioning to protect against further infestation. With such cleansing and restoration relapse will not occur in most cases.

Bacterial Polluters

In August 1992, two farm workers were exposed to poisonous gases when they entered a hog manure waste pit to repair a clogged pump. Overcome and unable to breathe, they quickly suffocated to death. Why? As the bacteria in the manure decomposed, they generated several toxic gases: methane, hydrogen sulfide, carbon dioxide, and ammonia. In combination, these gases can cause death both from oxygen deficiency and from the toxic effects of the gases in those who breathe it.[6]

To a lesser degree, the putrefactive colon flora produces the same toxins that killed the farm workers. Is it any wonder that many people are sick and dying before their natural time? A slow and invisible process is destroying their health from the inside.

Again, the biology works as follows: The pathogenic bacteria secrete toxins as a result of their metabolic action on specific foods. Some of these toxins in the colon are the gases that create discomfort, bloating, foul odors, inflammation, and disease. Toxins created by these putrefactive bacteria pass from the colon, through the portal vein to the liver, and then to the blood where they circulate throughout the body. When the liver is weakened or overwhelmed by toxins that it can no longer break down as a result, some of these toxins will enter the bloodstream.

TABLE 5.
Toxins Produced in an Unhealthy Colon[7]

Aminoethyl mercaptan	The by-product of decomposition of cysteine, a naturally occurring amino acid. Its presence exerts a very strong hypotensive effect.
Ammonia	A by-product of urea and protein decomposition, formed by certain bacterial species in the colon. Normally, ammonia is converted to urea. When this conversion fails to occur, ammonia causes neurological symptoms and may be involved with malignant transformation of cells.
Histamine	Formed from the decomposition of tryptophan, an amino acid, it can cause head congestion, headache, cardiac arrhythmia, nervous depression, lowered blood pressure, nausea, and collapse.
Hydrogen sulfide gas	A by-product of protein decomposition, this gas irritates the inner lining of the colon and can be as toxic as cyanide in comparable amounts. It can cause weakness, rapid pulse rate, nausea, and death.
Indole	A by-product of tryptophan decomposition. A diet high in meat consumption increases indole, sometimes referred to as indican. A normally functioning liver is able to detoxify indole.

Phenol or carbolic acid	A putrefactive by-product of tyrosine decomposition in the colon, causing necrosis (death of the tissues) of the gastrointestinal mucosa and liver cells.
Skatole	Another by-product of tryptophan decomposition, related to malabsorption syndrome and anemias. When in excess, skatole can circulate through the blood, resulting in foul odor emanating from the breath and stool. Skatole antagonizes acetylcholine and potassium.
Tyramine	A putrefactive by-product formed from the decomposition of the amino acid tyrosine and structurally similar to epinephrine. When it circulates in the bloodstream, it can raise blood pressure and cause central nervous system problems.

Even a healthy liver is unable to break down a small percentage of these toxins, such as phenol and skatole, which can then poison the nervous system.

In 1994, many people became seriously ill and a few died from consuming improperly cooked meat contaminated with *E. coli*. Nationwide awareness of the danger of pathogenic bacteria grew in response. In the colon, putrefactive bacteria, which can exist only in an alkaline pH, excrete gas. People frequently complain about flatulence (gas). Some gas may be due to poor digestion or eating wrong food combinations. This can usually be identified quickly because it is temporary and passes out of the colon readily. When gas is due to harmful bacteria overpopulating the colon, the smell is usually unpleasant, strong, and the gas is frequent. When the acidophilus colon flora is restored, there is no odorous gas.

Over the past 20 years, medical researchers have discovered that bacteria play a key role in many diseases, including cancer. The abnormal colon flora has been found to be directly linked to the formation of some human cancers. Researchers have found that bacteria in the colon modify substances they come in contact with and influence the human internal environment.[8] Data do suggest a correlation between an alkaline fecal pH, the composition of the colon microflora, and an increased risk of colon cancer.[9,10]

Around the turn of the nineteenth century, the fathers of contemporary medicine at the Pasteur Institute in Paris established that as flowing water eventually reaches the lowest level on land, so molecular toxins in the bloodstream flow to the weakest area in the system. Once toxic accumulation challenges a weak area, such as fatty breast tissue, tumors or cancer can result.[11] Everything is cause and effect.

In addition, many bacteria are found to be capable of modifying a "wide range of environmental chemicals and in particular intestinal bacteria can modify food additives ... [and] digestive secretions like bile salts and hormones. . . ."[12]

Strong evidence also points to a connection between both breast and colon cancer and colon bacteria.[13,14,15,16,17] Studies show that *E. coli* can synthesize a known carcinogen, ethionine.[18] *Clostridium paraputrificum* may be implicated in transforming bile acids into potential carcinogens.[19]

Researchers know that estrogens stimulate tumor growth, and some even state that certain forms of estrogens may actually cause tumors to develop.

There are several types of estrogens occurring naturally in the body. Of the three most important types of estrogen (estrone, estradiol, and estriol), estradiol is found to be the most stimulating to the breast tissue. In fact, it is 1,000 times more stimulating to the breast than estriol. Estradiol is also found to increase one's risk of breast cancer.[20]

What is not widely known, however, is that bacteria in the abnormal colon flora can produce estrogens and other carcinogens from biliary steroids and bile acids present in the colon.[21,22,23,24]

High-fat diets tend to increase the amount of biliary steroids found in the colon. The colon flora of people who eat high-fat diets contains a higher percentage of bacteria that can produce estrone and estradiol. These forms of estrogen are linked with tumor growth.[25]

Some bile acids have been shown to be carcinogenic, while others can be converted by bacterial action into potent carcinogens.[26] In 1994, a study found bile acids in breast cyst fluid that were proven to be of intestinal origin.[27]

Interestingly, the highest incidence of breast and colon cancers is found in developed nations, where diets are highest in fat and animal protein and lowest in cereal fibers.[28,29,30,31] Studies now also conclude that low fecal pH is more relevant in decreasing the incidence of colon cancer than the role of dietary fiber.[32]

Dietary factors have a great influence on and can promote either health or disease, not only through nutrition, but also by affecting the colon flora.[33,34,35,36] The type of bacteria contained in the colon has a profound impact on the level of our health

Questions and Answers

Q. *I have been told I have* Candida *and need to go on a cleansing regime and very restrictive diet. What do you think of this?*

A. It is absolutely essential to know if you actually have *Candida* before you treat yourself or go on any program. The only way to determine if you really have *Candida* is through a lab test given by your doctor. Many people go on radical diets which only weaken them, just because they think they have *Candida*.

Q. *Does Kyolic® liquid aged garlic have any effect against* Candida?

A. Kyolic® liquid is a special aged garlic product found in health food stores. Laboratory studies have found that Kyolic® liquid aged garlic (refer to Appendix B) eliminated *Candida* from the blood and kidneys of animals. It did so not by directly killing *Candida* but by stimulating the immune system, specifically by enhancing phagocyte function. The phagocytes eat harmful microorganisms. In this study it was found that Kyolic® stimulated the phagocytes which eliminated the yeast organisms from the body.[37]

According to Dr. Benjamin Lau, *Candida* organisms exist in two different forms. As part of the healthy colon flora, where they are in the minority, *Candida* exist in an oval-shaped, budding yeast form. It is only in an imbalanced state that *Candida* become elongated and invasive to the human host. Laboratory studies have shown that Kyolic® prevents *Candida* organisms from transforming into the invasive elongated form.[38] Certainly, these studies suggest that Kyolic® could be a useful adjunct to medical therapy for *Candida*.

Over the years, I have had many woman report relief

from vaginal infections and vaginal *Candida* by using a Kyolic® douche. They combine 1 teaspoon of liquid aged garlic with 1 pint of pure water and douche once daily until their symptoms are gone. They follow this with one douche of 1 tablespoon of whey mixed in with 4 capsules of Kyo-Dophilus® (refer to Appendix B) emptied into 1 pint of pure water. After this, they do not douche again unless necessary. The vagina, like the colon, needs to be maintained at a slightly acid pH and houses a natural acidophilus flora that must be maintained for health.

6

KEYS TO HEALTH: COLON AND LIVER

■

The liver is an important processing center in the body in charge of a multitude of functions that protect us from toxins and keep our organs running smoothly. A vital part of our immune system, the liver also breaks down toxins to be eliminated and nutrients to be absorbed by the body. The liver is involved with bile production, formation of plasma proteins, breakdown of worn-out blood cells, metabolism, and storage of nutrients. We will discuss the liver and see how a balanced colon flora benefits the liver and, therefore, the whole person.

In terms of ancient Chinese medicine, always a good source to refer to when considering health, the liver functions to ensure a smooth flow of energy and blood throughout the body. In Western medicine the liver plays a very similar role in the overall metabolism of the body, the storage of nutrients, and the continual processing of enormous amount of blood to sustain health and life.

In the process of digestion, nutrients such as carbohydrates, fats, and proteins are transported from the small intestine to the liver, which breaks them down into components that our cells can use for nourishment, growth and repair. The liver also carefully monitors and is responsible for the release of nutrients, particularly glucose, into the bloodstream for their use at a cellular level.

It is especially helpful to understand this process, in terms of colon health. Metabolism simply refers to the chemical processes that make it possible for our body's cells to continue living. Of course, a great deal of the chemical reactions that take place in cells are specifically geared to transform the energy stored in food for use in the body. In general, we receive about 45 percent of our energy from carbohydrates, among the two other food types we eat: protein and fat.[1] Because the source of our carbohydrates affects our energy levels and health, we will discuss this further. For its part, fat supplies almost 40 percent of the average American's energy needs, which in worldwide terms is quite high due to the excessive fat content in our standard diet. Ideally, the energy we take from fat should be half or less than half that amount, ranging between 15 and 20 percent. Protein is the primary nutrient the body uses for repair and maintenance of cells, organs, and organ systems. Three-quarters of bodily solids are composed of proteins.[2] As a result, the body uses protein for energy only as a last resort. The body gets almost 15 percent of its energy from protein, which it then breaks down into amino acids.

Liver

The liver is our storage house for energy. It stores energy by hoarding glucose. In the process of digestion, the body breaks down carbohydrates into simpler molecules, mostly glucose—the main sugar the body uses as fuel. The body uses glucose immediately for release of energy at the cellular level and it also stores glucose for later use in the form of glycogen. Although many cells can store glycogen, liver cells do so best, storing as much as 5 to 8 percent of their weight as glycogen, making the liver its main storage area. As energy is needed by the body, enzymes in the liver convert the stored glycogen back to glucose, which is then released into the bloodstream. This system is designed to keep a steady supply of nutrients in our bloodstream, so we can keep an even stream of energy throughout our days and nights.

In addition to processing glucose, other nutrients such as proteins and fats are transported from the small intestine to the liver. Here they are broken down further into components such as amino acids and lipids that cells can then use. There is no question that the liver's role in metabolizing and storing nutrients affects our sense of well-being and energy level on a day-to-day basis.

Continuing in its role as a major processing center, the liver is also the body's primary organ for detoxification. The liver breaks down toxins so they can be excreted from the body. At the same time, the liver functions as part of the immune system by filtering all the blood and lymph in the body. The liver is very permeable to fluids such as the blood and lymph, which flow freely through it. The liver expands and contracts, depending on the amount of blood it holds at any given time. In fact, the liver usually holds about one-tenth of the body's blood volume at any one time. Under certain disease conditions, it may expand to hold as much as one-quarter of the body's blood. Under stress, the veins of the liver can contract to hold as little as one-thirtieth of the body's blood.

The liver contains almost 50 percent of all macrophages in the body. Recall that macrophages are one of the most important cell types actively involved in the immune response. Their specific job is to defend against microorganisms and harmful chemicals. The macrophages in the liver are called Kupffer cells and are embedded in liver sinusoids, the large permeable capillaries that allow the Kupffer cells to cleanse the blood of bacteria and other contaminants. Otherwise, the liver receives toxins and microorganisms primarily from the digestive tract through the blood which empties into the liver through the portal vein. This is the link which helps us again understand clearly how an unhealthy colon affects the whole body and contributes to degeneration and disease.

Autointoxication

The New Shorter Oxford English Dictionary defines a toxin as "Any poisonous antigenic substance produced by or derived from micro-organisms, which causes disease when present at low concentration in the body."[3] Toxins are not the pathogens themselves, but are substances produced by the pathogens. Autointoxication is defined as a condition that results when poisonous substances are produced within the body.[4] Although not recognized officially by modern medicine, autointoxication can cause many diseases. Certainly, toxins can be produced within the body or introduced from without. Sources of external toxins include drugs, contaminated food, and pesticide ingestion or inhalation. Internally, the main source of toxins comes from an unhealthy colon.

In previous chapters, we have shown what happens when pathogens gain hold in an unhealthy colon. The secretions of these pathogenic microorganisms—whether bacteria, parasites, or other organisms—are toxins that cause varying amounts of damage to the host. These toxins can migrate to other sites in the body, causing autointoxication and, eventually, disease. Different factors will determine where disease manifests in the body, what symptoms will arise, and the various degrees of illness—depending on a person's immune system and overall health, as well as the strength and amount of the pathogen secreting toxins. Some pathogens are extremely virulent and can cause severe illness and death quite quickly, even in healthy people. Others, such as *Candida albicans* and most parasites, can exist for many years in a healthy person and take over when trauma or illness results in a weakened immune system. They can be present, showing no visible effects, for a long time until the balance is tipped in their favor and they begin to proliferate.

There are two main sources of toxins emanating from the colon. First, there are the by-products of unhealthy colon flora or other pathogens residing in the colon. Second, there is what results from the improper functioning of the ileocecal valve. Located between the end of the small intestine and the beginning of the large intestine, the ileocecal valve is a doorway that opens into the cecum at the lower part of the ascending colon. The valve opens only in one direction, preventing waste material from reentering the small intestine. In a very small number of people, the valve does not shut completely. In these cases, bacteria can be forced into the lower small intestine, the ileum, where food absorption is still taking place.[5] The presence of fecal material and bacteria in the ileum can contaminate the lymphatic system and bloodstream, as material from the ileum passes directly into these areas. Fortunately, only a small minority of people are known to suffer from this condition.

Just how do toxins produced in the colon affect the rest of the body? Toxins are transported, as a matter of course, from the colon through the portal vein to the liver. The health of the liver, bloodstream, and body is thus directly affected by the colon.

Blood circulates through the body in two kinds of blood vessels. The arteries carry fresh, oxygenated blood (red blood) from the heart to supply all the organs and tissues of the body. The veins carry waste materials away from the organs and tissues. Venous blood does not contain oxygen (that's why it is blue in color) and returns to the heart. From the heart, blood passes to the lungs, is reoxygenated, and becomes red blood again. This blood then reenters the heart before circulating once more through the arteries.

The superior and inferior mesenteric arteries carry fresh blood to the colon. Likewise, mesenteric veins carry blood, nutrients, and waste materials away from the colon. The inferior mesenteric vein carries blood away from the rectum, sigmoid colon, and descending colon. The superior mesenteric veins return blood from the small intestine, the cecum, and from the ascending and transverse portions of the colon. The inferior mesenteric vein empties into the splenic vein, which comes from the spleen. The splenic vein and superior mesenteric veins join to form the portal vein, which lies about level with the second lumbar vertebrae and passes upward into the liver.

Both nutrients and waste materials are carried into the liver from the portal vein along with various "toxic substances harmful to the tissues of the body."[6] Even in seemingly healthy people, hundreds of substances originating from the colon can escape across the colon's mucosal border. All of these need to be detoxified by the liver, presuming it is not already overloaded.[7]

The liver is constantly accumulating and distributing blood. It circulates about 1.5 liters of blood per minute and 70 percent of this blood flow arrives from the portal

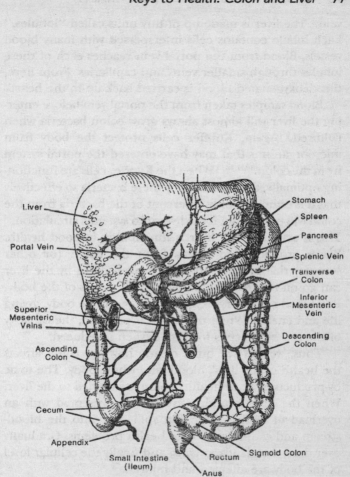

Liver

Portal Vein

Superior
Mesenteric
Veins

Ascending
Colon

Cecum

Appendix

Small Intestine
(Ileum)

Stomach

Spleen

Pancreas

Splenic Vein

Transverse
Colon

Inferior
Mesenteric
Vein

Descending
Colon

Sigmoid Colon

Rectum

Anus

Figure 5. Portal Vein System

vein.[8] The liver is made up of tiny units called "lobules." Each lobule contains cells interspersed with many blood vessels. Blood from the portal vein reaches each of these lobules through smaller veins and capillaries. From here, this deoxygenated blood is carried back up to the heart.

Blood samples taken from the portal vein before entering the liver will almost always grow colon bacteria when cultured.[9] Again, Kupffer cells protect the body from microorganisms that may have entered the portal system from the colon.[10,11,12,13] When the Kupffer cells are functioning optimally, they will destroy these bacteria so effectively that it is estimated only 1 percent of the bacteria from the colon will pass through the liver into systemic circulation.[14] This is assuming the liver is functioning in good health. Waste products and toxins from the colon (or other sources) that are not properly broken down by the liver can go on to affect the blood and all tissues of the body. Red blood cells carry oxygen throughout the body, giving life and energy. When the blood is polluted, the capacity of the red blood cells to carry oxygen is reduced.

Thus, we can see quite clearly how the colon affects the health of the liver, blood, and whole body. The toxic by-products of an unhealthy colon are carried to the liver. When the liver is under stress or is presented with an overload of toxins, these can spill over into the bloodstream and cause a variety of health problems. Gradually over time, the glands, organs, and finally the cellular level of the body are affected and injured.

This is why it is so important for anyone with health problems, especially liver problems, to have a clear, healthy colon which minimizes the toxic burden on the liver. In health, a minimum of toxins will flow from the colon, thus relieving the burden on the liver. When the colon is healthy and at a slightly acidic pH, nutrients from the colon enter the liver to be directed into the bloodstream.

However, even when a person's diet and colon pH are optimal, if the liver is still congested or weakened from being overwhelmed by toxins, the body will not function at top performance levels. As a result, even the best nutrition will be inadequate because a polluted or weakened system will not be able to properly assimilate foods essential for health. It's thus very important to clear and restore to health the liver and the colon *at the same time.*

Colon and Liver Cleansing

When you clean out your colon and liver, you gain immediate health benefits, especially in relation to toxins. With your colon and liver now much stronger and healthier, your other organs, tissues, and lymph nodes will wish to follow suit, ridding themselves of the toxins previously stored up within them. Quite simply, they will dump their toxins into the bloodstream for the liver to process and pass on for final elimination through the now healthy colon, kidneys, and bladder. For more details here, you may wish to refer to the next chapter, "Organs of Elimination."

There are some excellent products and herbs that work to cleanse and heal the liver very gently and effectively. Of importance here is specially aged, liquid garlic extract (refer to Appendix B for more clarification). Although some people may have trouble with raw garlic (it can irritate the stomach and aggravate the kidneys), they shouldn't have any problems with aged garlic extract. High in naturally occurring sulfur compounds that help to purify the system, aged garlic extract also contains cysteine compounds—themselves powerful antioxidants that benefit the liver and immune system. Studies have found that aged garlic extract helps to detoxify heavy metals as well, such as lead, mercury, copper, and aluminum.[15]

How can you tell though if your liver is having trouble detoxifying your system? Look at your eyes! The presence of dark circles under the eyes is a sure sign of liver trouble. Usually, adding a teaspoon of aged garlic to your daily diet for one to six months will solve the problem, and the dark circles will disappear. You should also know that the liver goes through a two-stage detoxification process. Phase one involves the breakdown of toxins into a simpler form that is usually, but not always, less toxic. In phase two, these compounds are complexed with sulfur and amino acids, then excreted from the body through the bile or urine. In the long term, consuming one or two bottles of aged garlic extract each year, along with a healthy program of foods and herbs, should be sufficient to clear up and revitalize your liver.

Time is also an element in cleansing the liver. For there is a best time to do this, and it occurs during spring. There is a reason for this. During winter months, as a response to the cold, the body concentrates its energy in the deep layers or core of the body. It does so to conserve energy and health. It is the same in the vegetable kingdom: a seed goes dormant as the frost, snow, or ice builds above it only to sprout and grow toward the warm light of spring. Likewise, the body's energy starts to push outward. It's a good idea to work with this natural flow of energy. As the body pushes energy and toxins from its deeper layers, using what it needs and eliminating what it doesn't, why not help it along? As ever, take some care in how you do this; know what you're doing and why. For example, we suggest that you consult with someone trained and experienced in Chinese herbal medicine and nutrition to help you design a liver program that will address your specific needs at this time of year.

Clear the Bloodstream

After clearing the colon and liver, your next step is to help the bloodstream clean itself. Because pollution in the bloodstream depletes the normal capacity for oxygen transfer between blood and tissue cells, a more general oxygen deficit in the body can occur. It's very much like trying to breathe the polluted air in our cities and coming up short of breath. With more pollutants in the air, there's less oxygen to take in. Fortunately, though, after you cleanse the colon and restore a slightly acid pH to it, the system starts to regain oxygen, releasing more energy, and returning the skin in many people to a healthy color almost immediately.

One ideal substance to help the bloodstream regain its normal capacity to transfer oxygen to tissues is chlorophyll in concentrated form. In fact, chlorophyll concentrate acts quite similarly to hemoglobin, the red pigment in blood. The only difference between the two concerns the mineral in the nucleus of the molecule: A chlorophyll nucleus contains copper while a hemoglobin nucleus contains iron. Chlorophyll helps remove toxins from the body, builds blood, renews tissues, and helps improve liver function. Refer to Appendix B for more information.

Exercise—Key to Health

Exercise is also important to keep the liver and colon healthy. Exercise that works the back thigh muscles assists the heart's pump and enhances blood circulation. Recall that blood carries nutrients to and toxins away from organs and tissues. Regular exercise helps the smooth flow of nutrients, energy, and blood through the body. Since the colon wall is composed of muscular tissue, exercise also helps to tone this important and little considered muscle while promoting good peristalsis and regular bowel movements. I have seen over three thousand clients, and those who exercise daily, even if it's just a walk, clearly have good peristalsis.

Lymph fluid bathes the tissues and acts as a drain system for the body. The lymphatic system has no internal pump and flows in only one direction. It is only through exercise that you can keep your lymph circulating properly to cleanse the system of toxins at a cellular level. About one-half to two-thirds of the lymph formed in the body comes from the liver.[16]

Liver circulation is aided by the action of the abdominal muscles and the diaphragm. As the diaphragm expands the chest, it compresses the abdominal cavity. The gentle compression of the liver with every breath aids the circulation of fluids through the liver. In addition to exercise, yogic breathing is an excellent way to promote liver circulation and health.

Swimming, too, comes into play here. Because it utilizes all the muscles and combines rhythmic breathing and stretching of the muscles, swimming is an excellent exercise. Bicycling, walking or jogging just 30 minutes daily is also very beneficial. Another exercise possibility is the trampoline. Using a small home trampoline only 10 to 15 minutes a day is sufficient to help circulate the lymph. A simple program of situps targets the abdominal muscles, which benefits the colon musculature and digestive system directly.

Our entire body is basically a filtration system. Our colon and liver are like the oil pan and oil filter in a car. We must ensure the filter is clean at all times to keep the engine running clean and well. To clear the liver without addressing the colon is like replacing the oil filter and not changing the oil.

Questions and Answers

Q. *What herbs are helpful for the liver?*

A. Because it is such a major organ, there are many approaches to support the liver. Herbs that help to clear the liver include dandelion, burdock, and chrysanthemum. These are cooling herbs to cleanse toxins from the liver. Outstanding herbs to protect and nourish the liver include milk thistle and Reishi mushrooms. They work to enhance liver function and can help to regenerate the liver. The best way to use herbs is in the form of a liquid tincture or tea. The liquid form of herbs is easily absorbed into the bloodstream. These herbs are usually all available at the health food store.

Q. *Are there vitamins and nutrients that help the liver?*

A. Specific nutrients such as lipoic acid, glutathione, and N-acetyl-cysteine work to protect and restore liver function. These are also powerful antioxidants that help the cells' ability to quench free radicals and eliminate them from the body.

Lipoic acid specifically helps regenerate the liver. All these nutrients work at the cellular level to increase efficient respiration and regeneration of cells. B vitamins help the liver by enhancing absorption, storage, and utilization of carbohydrates.

7

ORGANS OF ELIMINATION

■

A simple law of nature states that what goes in must come out. Everything we ingest is utilized by the body, stored in the body, or excreted. To maintain health, our two basic functions of digestion and elimination must perform well. We will discuss digestion in Chapter 11. Here we will come to understand the colon's central role and how it influences all the other organs of elimination.

Many Western health practices emphasize cleansing the body of toxins in order to regain health. Different methods are used to accomplish this including homeopathy, colon therapy, herbal medicine, and fasting. Fasting can actually be detrimental to our health because all the different toxins dumping into the system at once can weaken the body and cause long-term damage.

The Folly of Long Fasts

This true story of a 65-year-old client illustrates several reasons why fasting can be inappropriate. My client's livelihood required that he work in close proximity to harmful pesticides for over 30 years. On his own, this man decided he would benefit from a strict cleansing fast.

He began his regimen by consuming only distilled water for a few days. The following week, he drank only juice. He did well until the tenth day, when he began to feel weak and called a nutritionist for advice. She correctly instructed him to start eating soft foods, such as cooked vegetables, for nourishment and in order to slow the detoxification process. Although he followed her advice, he became weaker.

The nutritionist suspected that chemicals from his occupational exposure had been stored deep in his tissues. Owing to the fast, these chemicals were now being released into his bloodstream. Within ten more days, he became nervous, his speech was slurred, and his muscles began to cramp and stiffen, yet he continued this self-imposed, radical cleansing routine for two months, without ever consulting a health professional again.

At this time, he changed his routine to include much bed rest, a strict nutritious food intake, and light exercise. At the end of a year and a half, he gradually started to return to normal. His previously white teeth, however, had already turned brown, and his dentist couldn't whiten them. This shows how deeply he had stressed his system.

When an individual undertakes radical detoxification without understanding the mechanisms that affect our health, the results may be worse than doing nothing at all. In this example, the man threw his balance off completely by detoxifying too quickly. Because his system had compensated for the toxins within it, and especially for the toxins deep in his system, they went unnoticed prior to his strict fast.

Quite simply, fasting releases toxins stored in the body. In many people, the liver cannot keep pace nor is it able to deal with the newly released toxins effectively. The toxins are then thrown into the blood circulation. This is why a person can experience severe symptoms, as did the man in the example above.[1]

When chemicals and drugs stored in the tissues are dumped into the bloodstream, a person will very often reexperience their effects. Since a variety of chemicals may be released at the same time, the effects are unpredictable and may cause long-term damage. Our bodies are not meant to handle so many toxins all at once, let alone in a weakened, fasting state.

In this day and age, with widespread use of drugs of all types, pesticides, and other chemicals in the food chain, the human system is being challenged as never before in history. When someone goes on an extended fast, all these chemicals will suddenly dump into the bloodstream, causing immense discomfort and possibly overloading the system's capacity. Prolonged or excessive fasting throws more toxins into a situation that is already toxic. Continual fasting and cleansing further weaken the system, leaving it vulnerable to illness or pathogens.

Fasting was a much more straightforward process in simpler days. Historically, nature cure doctors used fasting, fruits, vegetables, and other cures drawn from nature to treat their clients. These doctors would fast clients for as many as 40 to 100 days. Leon Chaitow, a prominent naturopath and osteopath in England, states this cannot be done anymore. As he puts it: If we put somebody on a long fast who's had steroids, antibiotics or fifteen other strong drugs, God knows what's in their fatty tissues and what will come flooding back into the system. . . . We can't expect the same results anymore. We've changed the organism so we must modify the approach.[2]

Leading health professionals no longer recommend

extended fasts.[3,4] Experts state that fasts of a few days at a time are the longest that should be undertaken. If a fast longer than this is indicated, it is best done under supervision of a qualified professional with experience in this area. I have found fasting to be unnecessary in almost all cases. There is certainly no need for detoxifying the body to be a dramatic or traumatic event, as it often has been in the old-school tradition of long-term, radical fasts. Do not experiment with your health. It is not worth it.

Balanced Cleansing

Before undertaking any type of cleansing program, we need to assess several factors. First, there must always be a balance between nourishing and cleansing the person. Nourishing means to provide the body with energy to perform its daily functions, the work the person needs to do, and additional energy to go through the healing process. Whether the emphasis is more on nourishing or more on cleansing will depend on the basic constitution and overall health of the person. If he or she is strong and healthy, the emphasis can be on cleansing. If he or she is weak or depleted with low energy, the emphasis will be on providing nourishment and support for the system. In this case, cleansing will proceed more slowly and more gently. If too much of a detoxifying treatment is given to a weak person, he often suffers ill effects, including some compromise to his immune system.

Remember that the body does its own housecleaning and at its own rate. When a person is strong and healthy, she will eliminate toxins quickly and efficiently alongside the process of digestion. In a weak person, the body does not have enough energy to digest or eliminate efficiently.

When properly nourished and optimally functioning, the body can follow its own natural wisdom about how and when to eliminate any toxins. Like a good housekeeper, it knows the best time to do light cleaning or heavy cleaning. The body loses this wisdom when it is unhealthy or overwhelmed with pollution, but regains it in health.

Toxins that have accumulated over a lifetime cannot be eliminated in a day, a week, or even a month. In general, health professionals believe that it takes one month for each year of life to effect a positive change. In fact, it often takes much longer, depending on the person and his or her constitution and circumstances.

We know that when excessive amounts of toxins are released into circulation, the body has a very difficult time eliminating them and in counteracting a parallel suppression of the immune system. In traditional Chinese medicine, when the toxins are powerful and the person is deficient or weak, the primary consideration is to build up the strength and immunity of the individual, not the opposite. In this case, cleansing is inappropriate and will only further weaken the person, putting at risk the chance for full recovery of health.

Modern scientific research confirms that an undernourished, depleted person is less able to eliminate certain toxins. With proper nourishment comes improved excretion of toxins.[5,6] The good health and stamina of a person is what keeps him from being overwhelmed by most toxins or pathogens. A person can clear himself of toxins, and do so at his own pace, avoiding thereby a more dramatic and possibly traumatic cleansing regimen.

Alternative approaches that cleanse the body without fasting are available. The ancient Chinese medicine practitioners understood the necessity of clearing toxins and pathogens out of the body. Licensed acupuncturists, well trained in Chinese herbal medicine, can skillfully adjust the interplay between cleansing and nourishing an individual.

Organs of Elimination

There is a third key factor in cleansing the body effectively. The organs of elimination must be in top working condition. European doctors, for example, commonly emphasize the importance of making sure that the organs of elimination are working well *before* undertaking any cleansing program. They use the term "emunctory" in this regard, which means "a part of the body that serves to cleanse it or get rid of waste products."[7] Before beginning any kind of cleansing, make sure your organs of elimination are perfectly healthy.

If the emunctories are not open, then the body will not be able to eliminate the toxins dumped into the bloodstream from the fatty tissues and organs. It's just like throwing your garbage into the trash can. It's there all right, but now you have to take the trash can outside for the garbage truck to haul it to the dump. If you don't, your house will pile up high with trash with all its unsanitary aftereffects. Toxins that are not eliminated from the body will redeposit somewhere else in the body, creating a whole new set of problems for you. In Europe, they have a colorful term to describe the movement of toxins around in the body: They call it the "toxic Ping-Pong effect."

The major emunctories in the body are the liver, kidneys, urinary bladder, lungs, skin, and colon. All of them must be open and working at optimum levels for a healing program to be effective. The colon is the central and most important emunctory to be addressed in any detoxification or healing program. When the colon is clear, it takes the burden off all the other emunctories. When the colon is not functioning correctly, this has a domino effect on other organs of elimination. We will go through each emunctory system to understand how this can be true.

Liver

In the last chapter, we saw how an unhealthy colon flora generates toxins that are carried to the liver through the portal vein. When the liver becomes overloaded or is already not functioning correctly, other areas are affected as well. Toxins will then pass into the bloodstream and from there be deposited in the organs, tissue, and cells of the body. Restoring the colon to optimal health relieves the burden on the liver. Dark circles under the eyes reflects this and shows a lack of oxygen transfer in the system. A motor with a dirty oil filter does not perform at its best, nor does a body whose filtering system is clogged with toxins. Chronic fatigue and many other serious diseases result from a polluted bloodstream that lacks oxygen.

Kidneys and Urinary Bladder

Next in line, the kidneys become challenged and toxins move into the bladder. Often the first indication that the kidneys are under duress is puffiness under the eyes.[8] Other concerns arise here as well. When a woman has recurrent bladder infections, she needs to take some care with hygiene habits to avoid further contamination. She should never allow fecal material, for instance, to come in contact with the vaginal area. If personal hygiene habits are not an issue and the infections continue, then she might consider

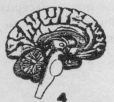

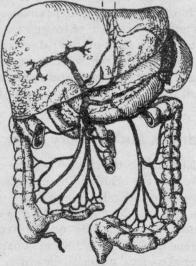

5

The kidney and urinary
bladder are also
overwhelmed by excess
toxins. This can contribute
to kidney problems and
chronic bladder infections.

4

Toxins can affect
the brain and nervous
system, causing
headaches and other
symptoms. Some toxins
can cross the blood-
brain barrier.

3

Toxins leave the liver and enter the bloodstream.
They flow through the body, affecting
the weakest body areas.

2

Toxins are not
completely broken
down by the already
challenged liver.

1

Alkaline colon pH.
Toxins formed in the
colon flow through the
mesenteric veins,
into the portal vein,
and then into the liver.

Figure 6. Unhealthy Colon Function

1

Predominance and maintenance of healthy colon flora with a slightly acidic pH ensures an insignificant amount of toxins are formed in the colon. Portal system transport from colon to liver consists mainly of nutrients formed by the lactobacteria flora.

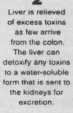

2

Liver is relieved of excess toxins as few arrive from the colon. The liver can detoxify any toxins to a water-soluble form that is sent to the kidneys for excretion.

3

Normal excretion of water-soluble substances through the kidney and urinary bladder.

Figure 7. Healthy Colon Function

colon health as a contributing factor. The colon is very close to the bladder and toxins from the colon will directly and indirectly affect the bladder. Once the colon is restored to its proper health, however, the bladder will be able to regain its own normal functions—if it has not degenerated too far.

Dr. Empringham, whom we previously noted as an early leader in colon research, described the presence of indican in urine as a sign of colon toxicity. Although the urine test for indican is rarely used today, medical professionals may want to consider reevaluating its validity. I offer the following story from Dr. Empringham, published originally in 1940, as an important side note here.

> The difference between the old and new methods of urinalysis is very great. For example, in [America] little importance is paid to indican. This toxin comes from residues decomposing in the bowels. It is found in the urine of almost every civilized person. Therefore, formerly, doctors thought indican natural. In America most laboratory reports say, "Indican—Normal." But we now know this poison is *never normal*. It is usual but not normal, natural, or necessary.[9]

Empringham found that when the native flora is restored to the colon, a person's urinalysis will show no trace of indican.

Lungs and Skin

The health of the colon has a direct effect on the lungs and skin. Whenever the skin or lungs are in an unhealthy state, the colon must be cleared and its natural flora restored before a person can regain health. Recall that when the colon is overloaded with toxins, these are dumped into the liver; when the liver is overburdened, it cannot process these same toxins, which are then dumped into the bloodstream. Now some of these toxins will deposit in the body tissues and some will seek another avenue of elimination, such as the skin and lungs.

The lungs breathe in air, extracting the oxygen that we need to live, which then circulates through the bloodstream. Waste materials are also expelled from the lungs when we exhale. When the lungs are overburdened, conditions such as asthma and other breathing difficulties can develop.

The skin is porous and secretes waste material through sweat. Acne, psoriasis, eczema, and other skin conditions are a sure sign of an underlying cause of a toxic colon that is not eliminating waste correctly.

Summary

We can now review the cycles of health and disease. Healthy people are strong with an abundance of free-flowing energy. They awake refreshed after a good night's sleep. They are efficient processors, assimilating necessary nutrients and eliminating toxins at a rate that ensures their system stays clean. Weak people do not assimilate nutrients well and toxins constantly accumulate in their system because their rate of elimination is slow and inefficient. They wake up in the morning feeling tired and sluggish. In today's world, because of the high amount of toxins we are exposed to in our air and food supply, the elimination organs are constantly at work and often unable to keep up with the demand placed on them.

When we cannot excrete toxins regularly and efficiently, they fall back to or remain in the body's tissues. Here the toxins cause degeneration and, eventually, disease. Usually they will deposit at sites which are the person's weakest areas, according to his genetic or constitutional weaknesses.

In all health programs, the colon needs to be addressed first. To attempt detoxification before addressing the colon is like giving your engine a carburetor flush and not draining the oil pan. Restoring the colon flora ensures optimal elimination. At the same time it relieves the toxic burden on the liver, kidneys, urinary bladder, lungs and skin, allowing them to eliminate at an optimal rate. This, in turn, relieves the amount of toxins circulating in the blood and lymph. When toxins are cleared from the blood and lymph, they will not deposit in the tissues and organs of the body. Keep your house clean and it will last a long time. It's about time we pay as much attention to what goes out as to what we're taking in. The first step in any healing therapy must be to restore the colon and open the emunctories so the body can clear toxins out of the body effectively.

Questions and Answers

Q. *Isn't psyllium helpful to promote colon health?*
A. No. And here's why.

One of the most widely used cleansers is psyllium. It is estimated that 4 million people use psyllium daily. In the past ten years, as people have sought to resolve their mounting colon problems, psyllium has become popular. When allowed to sit in a glass of water, psyllium turns into a thick, slimy, gelatinous substance. It absorbs forty times its weight in water!

To consider psyllium's effect here, remember that the colon is an absorption chamber. In the healthy system, when food residues empty through the ileocecal valve into the cecum, the residue is in a soft, liquid form. As the absorption process continues, the residue travels through the five-foot length of colon and the feces become more dry and solid. Water and electrolytes are reabsorbed back into the body. Psyllium can cause too much water absorption in the colon, thereby contributing to fecal impaction.

In a recent study, 24 healthy men over the age of 18 were given psyllium to test its cholesterol-lowering effect. These men had normal body weight, no disease, and were not taking any medications. The men reported the following adverse effects from ingesting psyllium: lower intestinal gas, indigestion, abdominal cramping, rectal pain, and diarrhea.[10]

I have seen many psyllium users complain of having no elimination for seven to ten days along with fatigue, lower back pain, constipation, and gas. They were no less than astonished to learn that what they thought was their top-notch cleanser had actually worsened their condition. Thirty percent of my scheduled appointments are made by people who have taken psyllium in some form. In small amounts, psyllium may be beneficial for a few people when used sparingly, but when used regularly or over the long term, it is a severe impediment to colon health.

The professional athlete who sought my services for an emergency appointment is a classic example of the psyllium syndrome. He was in his mid-thirties and had begun to ingest psyllium daily (1 tablespoon in 8 ounces of water, increasing consumption by 1 tablespoon per day) to clean his colon for better athletic performance. Previously, he had regular elimination every day. During the time he began ingesting psyllium, he made no dietary changes.

By the fifth day, he was ingesting 5 tablespoons of psyllium and had experienced no elimination. He assumed he needed more psyllium. He was experiencing severe back pain when he came slowly walking into my office. Seventy-five minutes into the colon hygiene procedure, 10 inches of solid psyllium mass began to move out of his colon. His relief was pronounced and he declared that he had no idea what he could have done to remove the problem on his own. Please note that there is no psyllium in breast milk.

Q. *What about using bentonite to promote colon health?*
A. Bentonite is a rock composed of clay minerals that has strong powers of absorption. Chemically, it is known as hydrated aluminum silicate[11] and is marketed in a powder or liquid form. Insoluble in water, it will swell to about 12 times its size when added to water.

People use bentonite because of claims that it cleanses the colon and pulls out all toxins, eliminating them from the body. Since bentonite has an alkaline pH, it leaves the colon in an alkaline condition, ripe for invasion by harmful microorganisms. Thus, use of bentonite cannot contribute to lasting colon health.

Q. *I have seen pictures of hardened, black masses several feet long, supposedly evacuated from the colon and often still in the shape of the colon. What is this about?*
A. In the past 25 years, these sensational pictures of so-called impactions in the colon have circulated throughout the health field. It has been stated that the fecal matter becomes encrusted on the colon wall and forms a solid mass of black matter that must be shed, much as a snake sheds its skin.

These pictures have caused fear and uneasiness in the

public. A person whose colon was near this type of condition would more likely be found in the obituary column than at a cleansing retreat. Most of the pictures of colon impactions are from people who have allegedly gone through rigorous cleansing programs before eliminating the black encrustations. Such programs included ingesting substances such as psyllium and bentonite. My theory is that using these substances possibly contributes to the formation of encrustations if, in fact, they exist at all. When the colon is already filled with alkaline, putrefactive waste, added bulk such as psyllium and bentonite can actually make the situation worse.

If you consult gastroenterologists who use fiber optic cameras in the colon, you will be told that they rarely, if ever, see anything as extreme as portrayed in these pictures. Never have I seen anything like this in my years of experience with colon hygiene.

8

AGING AND MENTAL HEALTH: THE COLON CONNECTION

∎

Let us return to the analogy of the automobile and the human body. Race cars maintained in excellent condition can run smoothly for years and achieve speeds of 200 miles per hour. Why? Because they are balanced and clean inside. The oil that goes up into the motor and circulates through the oil filter is not challenged with dirty oil. The exhaust is not impacted with waste and the cars are immaculately maintained, inside and out. All that moves, from the microcosm to the macrocosm, man to machine, undergo processes of intake or ingestion, combustion or digestion, exhaust or elimination. In all human or mechanical processes, cleanliness facilitates correct function. Disease can exist only in a proper medium. A healthy soil grows a healthy plant. By changing the medium to normal, starting from the foundation up, there should be no disease. This foundation is the colon.

Time Alone Does Not Make Us Old

Professor Metchnikoff, whom we discussed earlier as a pioneer in colon health, suggested we should live much longer than we do and explains why we do not. According to Metchnikoff, the average life span of civilized human beings is shorter than nature intended, and science may someday enable humanity to maintain youthfulness for a much longer time.

While at the University of Odessa, Dr. Metchnikoff became a student and follower of Owen, a comparative anatomist. Owen found the colons of many adults to be filled with trillions of harmful, putrefactive bacteria, generating toxic by-products. He did not find this condition in healthy animals. Owen attributed the failure of humans to live to a ripe old age to his finding of intestinal toxemia.

Apparently this was the clue that prompted Metchnikoff to consider the relationship between colon health and longevity. He soon became fascinated with prolonging the human life span in this regard. One of Metchnikoff's favorite theories, in fact, focused on the relationship between the poisons secreted by certain bacterial species in the colon and senility.[1]

The body is composed of trillions of cells. Each is a complete entity that breathes, eats, drinks, and excretes waste. At the end of a few days, weeks, or months, depending on the type of cell, it dies. Each of these microscopic living cells gives birth to a successor before it expires. As a result, our bodies are in continual flux. Little by little, every day we die; just as gradually and continuously, every moment, cell by cell, we are being reborn. About every seven years, every cell in our body has been replaced. We are a new person!

What is the cause of those changes we attribute to age? What is the cause of the phenomenon we call "natural death"? This is one of the most profound questions of biology. The answer is that, before our cells generate successors, they are continually poisoned and sometimes destroyed by unchecked toxins circulating in the bloodstream. Although this destruction of cells is a natural process, it is too often accelerated in modern society.

Sometimes the cells are replaced by dead matter instead of by new cells. In terms of the arterial system, we call this "arteriosclerosis," or "hardening of the arteries." Our blood vessels lose their natural elasticity as cells are replaced with inorganic mineral salts, fat, or other materials. As a result of this accumulation inside the vessels, the blood vessel's diameter decreases. Because of this smaller passageway, the heart must work harder to maintain circulation. While these symptoms are spoken of as "normal" responses to increased age, in truth, they are not. The number of years we have lived has nothing to do with degenerative changes due to an unhealthy lifestyle and diet. Within an unhealthy colon the toxins that develop there will stress an already overburdened liver, spill into the bloodstream, and affect other areas of the body.

Many people are not tired from overwork but rather think they are overworked because the labor they previously enjoyed has now become fatiguing. This is a condition of toxic fatigue. Normal fatigue is quickly cured by rest, but resting will not relieve a toxic condition. If one feels tired when arising after eight hours of sleep, the cause can be found in the toxins retained during sleep in the liver, heart, kidneys, and colon.

Putrefactive bacteria, multiplying in the colon, generate toxins that leak into the system through absorption. Gradually, over time, every gland, organ and cellular tissue of the human body is injured. According to Metchnikoff, this is the cause of most of the changes we falsely attribute to aging alone. Toxins stored in the body will eventually bring on almost every kind of degenerative disease, cutting our natural lifetime approximately in half.[2,3]

Vegetarians and the Toxic Colon

Many vegetarians believe they are free of toxins because they eat no meat and have a good diet. This is not necessarily true. A healthful diet alone will not correct an unhealthy colon flora. It is like strewing the best-quality seeds on the poorest of soils—nothing will happen. As we now know, many vegetarians also have toxic colons.

Amino acids, the basic components of protein, are found in all cells of living tissue and form the building blocks of all cells in our body. Even vegetarians have protein substances arriving in their colon, which can cause problems when the colon flora is already unbalanced. This is illustrated in the following story told by Dr. Empringham. Substitute the words "protein" or "amino acids" where he dramatically says "meat" and the picture becomes clearer.

"What is the matter with me?" said a patient the other day. "I have been ailing a long time, but no one seems able to find out what is wrong."

"Your trouble comes from meat," I remarked. "The analysis we have made proves that poisons are continually seeping into your blood from dead flesh decomposing in your colon."

The man laughed and said, "Meat! You think my troubles are caused by meat! Why, I have not eaten a morsel of meat for 30 years—nothing but fruits and vegetables.''

I said, "Yes, I know. you gave this information to the physician who took your history the day you came to see us. Nevertheless, your excreta contains meat. This would not matter, but unfortunately, your colon is cursed with putrefactive bacteria generating virulent toxins from your refuse."

Of course, there is nothing unusual about the colon residues containing meat. That is true of every human being, including those who live exclusively on fruits and vegetables. Even excreta from sheep, cows, and rabbits that eat nothing but grass contain meat. This is because the body of every creature consists of billions of microscopic cells, and every minute some of these cells that die are swept into the colon. Of course, these dead cells are perfectly harmless if they do not come in contact with putrefactive bacteria.[4]

Allergies

The toxins emanating from the abnormal colon flora appear to be directly related to food allergies, which are very widespread nowadays. Allergies are generally recognized as the system reacting inappropriately to certain foods or other substances. This happens because the body is overloaded with toxins. With the liver unable to function correctly, the bloodstream is polluted and low in oxygen.

In nearly 50 percent of the people I see, I have found reductions in food allergies after they eliminated the fecal material that accumulated in their system and reestablished a healthy colon flora. In all allergies, the colon must be addressed as a prime source of internal pollution.

Mental Health

The inability to function well in society is not a new manifestation. In 1929, N. W. Kaiser, M.D., reported his studies concerning the relationship between colon hygiene and mental disorders. In his report, he cited many other doctors who contributed to this field of research.

Dr. Kaiser considered constipation to be a probable cause of many obscure psychoses and to be responsible for such symptoms as apathy, irritability, melancholia, mania, and in some extreme cases, even suicidal inclinations.[5] The following study is from a test of mental patients with constipation at Toledo State Hospital, Ohio, performed in 1930.[6] The purpose of testing was to determine if constipation was the causative factor in mental problems or if mental problems were the cause of constipation.

In this study, constipation was defined as relative to the time required to eliminate barium meal. According to most medical authorities, the normal time to eliminate barium meal taken orally is between 36 and 48 hours. When elimination from the colon exceeds 48 hours, it is considered constipation.

Eighty percent of the 70 patients tested required more than 48 hours to eliminate the barium meal from their colon. One female manic-depressive patient required an amazing 240 hours before the barium meal was entirely eliminated.

These patients were given several colon hygiene water treatments. The mental conditions of many patients improved so greatly as a result that they were released from the mental hospital. However, some of these patients returned because of relapse, which is no surprise since nothing was done to reestablish the slightly acid pH and normal colon flora.

Dr. Kaiser's ideas were scoffed at by others, and as a result, his work went largely unnoticed. If we consider the connections between the unhealthy colon flora, an alkaline colon, and the toxins that circulate as a result of faulty elimination, Dr. Kaiser's ideas do not seem at all implausible. In addition, many toxins created in the putrefactive colon are capable of crossing the blood-brain barrier and have known mental effects. (Refer to Table 5 in Chapter 5 for more clarification here.) For example, histamine can cause nervous depression and tyramine can cause central nervous system problems. Skatole antagonizes acetylcholine, which is important in brain function and nerve signal transmission.

In 1930, the Royal Society of Medicine of Great Britain held a meeting on intestinal toxemia. Sixty leading physicians attended. It was reported that constipation caused accentuated mental symptoms such as melancholia, irritability, mania, and suicidal tendencies. Physically, a long string of degenerative diseases was also reported as arising from constipation.[7]

Why was this initial research discontinued when it showed a possible cause to major worldwide health problems? Currently, a few researchers are rediscovering the colon connection. A recent article by Jeffrey Bland, Ph.D. in chemistry, stated there are possible links (in combination with other factors) between colon-produced pathogens, the liver's detoxifying ability, and Parkinson's disease, Alzheimer's disease, and even schizophrenia.[8]

When the liver, the primary organ of detoxification in the body, is overwhelmed, toxins circulate in the body. A study of brain-injured children in Philadelphia, Pennsylvania, found many of them to have impaired colon and liver function. A direct connection was made between toxins originating in the colon that overloaded the liver and had an adverse effect on brain chemistry.[9]

In all cases, the weakest areas of the body are affected first and foremost. These weaknesses may be inherited or acquired during the wear and tear of life. After the passage of time, other sites may become affected as well. Depending on the type of damage that has occurred and its location, modern medicine can offer a diagnosis, labeling the disease process that has now set in. The essential area that must be addressed is the foundation of our healthy colon flora

Questions and Answers

Q. *Do mental and emotional stress affect the colon?*

A. Yes. Stress can cause the lower left descending colon, called the sigmoid flexure, to become spastic, cause dry constipation, and upset the colon. In some cases, relaxation can relieve the spasm. Many studies show the effect of emotions and stress on the entire digestive process. When a person is angry, upset, or under stress, he or she can neither digest nor assimilate food properly. This, in turn, affects the colon, which becomes burdened with improperly digested substances. Relaxation, meditation, breathing, yoga, and biofeedback can all help relieve stress and enhance colon health.

THE MISSING LINK: SETTING THE RECORD STRAIGHT

■

Acidophilus is considered synonymous with colon health. While this is true, there are many misconceptions about how to choose a good-quality acidophilus product and how to use it correctly. Unfortunately, marketing information has superseded scientific research, leading to much confusion.

Laypeople and health practitioners alike consider acidophilus supplementation to be the panacea for colon problems and postantibiotic care. Many holistic practitioners prescribe acidophilus supplements or yogurt for their patients after a course of antibiotics, although there is no scientific basis for doing so. There are many reasons why oral ingestion of acidophilus is not effective, however, as we shall see.

Mission Impossible

Health professionals and laypeople alike are under the misconception that oral ingestion of acidophilus achieves long-term colonization in the colon. If human beings could take acidophilus supplements orally to replenish their colon flora, there would be no life as we know it because it would mean the protective mechanism of the stomach was not functioning correctly. The concentrated stomach acids inactivate microorganisms ingested on food to prevent their entering any further into the human system.

Nonetheless, almost everyone is under the illusion that we need only to ingest one of the multitude of available acidophilus products. Presto! A few billion beneficial bacteria will then overcome some two pounds (or about one-third of the total fecal weight) of pathogenic bacteria in the alkaline colon, transform the pH to normal, and maintain normal pH from that moment on. If this were so, millions of consumers would have experienced an end to their suffering and there would have been no impetus for me to develop the scientific protocol that achieves what oral ingestion cannot. I have not found any data proving that implantation of the colon is achieved through taking acidophilus products orally. In fact, all the research I have seen clearly points to the opposite conclusion. Taking acidophilus orally cannot possibly replenish a damaged colon flora in an alkaline colon.

For example, in a 1984 study two strains of human *L. acidophilus* in milk were administered to individuals with no evidence that the intestine was permanently colonized with these strains.[1] A similar result was seen in a study that showed implantation of human *L. acidophilus* did not occur in the gastrointestinal tract of healthy men who orally ingested high doses.[2]

How will acidophilus survive the digestive tract where they are exposed to extreme acid conditions in the stomach and highly alkaline conditions in the healthy small intestine? If any do survive, they will then be faced with the unhealthy, alkaline colon dominated by putrefactive bacteria. They will be outnumbered and overwhelmed by the resident pathogens and yeasts of the alkaline colon. It is like sending a few Boy Scouts to fight a major war in a hazardous environment where the enemy already commands the territory. Let's follow their journey through the digestive tract.

Danger Zone 1: Stomach Acids

Digestive juices in the stomach are normally in the very acid pH range of 1.5 to 3.0. By definition, acidophilus will thrive only in a slightly acid environment, in the specific pH range of 4.5 to 6.4. Their growth stops when the acid pH of 4.0 to 3.6 is reached, depending on the species and strain.[3]

The following study is from promotional material distributed to consumers by Kovac Laboratories, Inc. around 1980. Kovac Laboratories had been in business more than 40 years and pioneered the first human-source liquid *L. acidophilus* sold in health food stores. An independent laboratory tested several brands of *L. acidophilus* drinks in a simulated stomach fluid with a pH of 1.2, the theoretical acidity at which humans digest protein. The initial shock of exposure to pH 1.2 killed from 40 to 70 percent of the acidophilus bacteria immediately. The loss after an additional 30 minutes was an additional 10 percent.[4]

Morning Star Laboratories, Inc. in Simi Valley, California, did the following experiment. They placed two strains, *L. acidophilus* and *B. bifidum*, in separate solutions of normal stomach acid for 30 minutes. None survived the stomach's strong hydrochloric acid that serves to break down certain foods and to kill microorganisms ingested with foods.[5]

In infants, these strong stomach acids are not yet active, allowing the *B. bifidum* in mother's milk to pass through

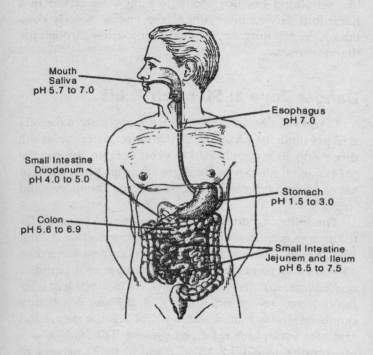

Mouth
Saliva
pH 5.7 to 7.0

Esophagus
pH 7.0

Small Intestine
Duodenum
pH 4.0 to 5.0

Stomach
pH 1.5 to 3.0

Colon
pH 5.6 to 6.9

Small Intestine
Jejunem and Ileum
pH 6.5 to 7.5

Acidophilus growth thrives in optimum range: pH 4.5 to 6.4

Acidophilus growth ceases at: pH 3.6 to 4.0

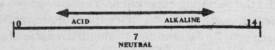

|0   ← ACID   ALKALINE →   14|
7
NEUTRAL

Figure 8. Acidophilus Growth pH Relative to Digestive pH

unharmed. While other bacteria can also pass through an infant's stomach unharmed, the *B. bifidum* acts as a protective barrier in the colon. In adults who are depleted or chronically ill, the stomach acids are deficient and may allow passage of the beneficial acidophilus as well as harmful microorganisms.

Danger Zone 2: Alkaline Small Intestine

If a few acidophilus bacteria do manage to escape annihilation by stomach acid, they are confronted with bile and other alkaline digestive secretions in the small intestine. Bile has an antibacterial effect and is responsible for the low transit numbers of bacteria in the healthy small intestine.[6] Pancreatic juice, which is secreted in the upper small intestine to aid digestion, has a pH range of 8.4 to 8.9. Other small intestinal secretions are in the alkaline range of 7.5 to 8.0. If acidophilus could live in an alkaline environment, they would be called "alkadophilus"!

Danger Zone 3: Unhealthy, Alkaline Colon

People take acidophilus because their colon is unhealthy. This means their colon is in an alkaline condition, with a majority of putrefactive bacteria. Even if a few acidophilus were to make it to the colon, it is like sowing seeds on unfertilized, unhealthy soil with the wrong pH. There will simply be no germination because it is not possible. Space in the colon is limited and the predominant, pathogenic microorganisms are not going to give up their established territory.[7] In order for the acidophilus to be able to tip the scales under these conditions, the scales must already be in their favor. They will be able to establish only in a colon that is already slightly acid. If the colon is already in good health with an acid pH, there is no need for acidophilus to be taken, because those already in the colon will thrive and multiply on their own.

Replenishing the Acidophilus Flora

If acidophilus supplements will not reestablish the healthy colon flora, then what will? Thanks to my experience and research I have found two procedures that will effectively reacidify the colon and restore the natural colon flora. One is by providing a food that will both acidify the colon and provide nutrients for the remaining acidophilus latent in the colon. This will stimulate their growth and proliferation. Most people can reestablish their beneficial colon flora within 3 to 8 weeks simply by including 3 to 6 tablespoons of edible-grade sweet dairy whey in their daily diet. (Refer to Appendix B for more information.)

If the colon is not normalized by about 8 weeks, this indicates the need for more direct action. Very often, the acidophilus flora has been severely damaged due to overuse of antibiotics or any of the other factors already discussed.

Webster Implant Technique™

A postantibiotic method is absolutely necessary to reimplant and reestablish the lost beneficial colon flora. The method I have developed involves application of whey enemas to gently clear and acidify the colon, followed by implanting a specific human strain of acidophilus culture in order to jump-start the colon's own acidophilus colony. The Webster Implant Technique™ (WIT) restores the acidophilus flora when it has been severely depleted. It duplicates breastfeeding in the adult colon.

This procedure should be standard after heavy therapeutic rounds of antibiotics or other medications, surgery, and other procedures known to destroy acidophilus either by direct action on the bacteria or through alkalinizing the colon, which would make it impossible for the acidophilus to live.

The process of caring for your colon health is similar to gardening. A healthy garden will be free of pests or major problems because everything is in balance and harmony. A good gardener knows the importance of nutrient availability and soil pH to assure good plant growth. When preparing a garden, the soil must first be tilled, loosened, and freed of major weed growth that will prevent crops from growing. Then nutrients can be added to the soil to nourish the plants and ensure correct soil pH for plant growth.

Even in an alkaline colon dominated by putrefactive bacteria, there may be a few surviving acidophilus, though they are rendered ineffective by being proportionately in the minority. If these survivors are provided with four factors, then these native acidophilus may be able to multiply and reestablish their predominance in the colon.

The four factors are:

1. Elimination of toxins and accumulated fecal matter from the colon. This is like weeding your garden.
2. Reestablishment of a slightly acid environment in

the colon to prepare the soil for the growth and proliferation of an acidophilus flora.

3. In a case of severely damaged flora, a rectal implant of a human-strain acidophilus with sufficient viability and high count is necessary. (Refer to Appendix B for more clarification here.) This is like planting seeds.

4. Proper food for nourishment to support the growth and proliferation of the acidophilus. This food is edible-grade, sweet dairy whey. This is like fertilizing your garden.

It is very important that the colon be cleared and acidified all the way to the cecum, so a reservoir of acidophilus can be reestablished there to ensure long-term results. In most people, using whey orally on a daily basis will both acidify the colon and promote the growth of the acidophilus that are latent in the colon. Step 3 is essential only when the colon flora is severely damaged.

Bacteria multiply by a process called fission, which is a method of cellular division. One bacterium divides to form two. When these two bacteria divide again, four are formed. Thus, bacteria grow at a geometric rate. Every 20 minutes a normal bacterium divides into two. In just 24 hours, this one bacterium is capable of becoming 17 million bacteria. Both alkaline- and acid-producing bacteria multiply in this manner, one toward health, the other toward disease. This natural law makes it imperative to maintain the normal acidophilus flora and acid pH in the colon.

Enemas

Traditionally in America, people have used enemas and water colonics as methods to cleanse the colon. Cleansing of the colon using enemas has been recorded since ancient times in Egypt, Arabia, Africa, Hawaii, India, and China. This procedure was considered important for physical health. Hippocrates, who is called the "Father of Medicine," used both enemas and suppositories containing various ingredients. He recommended enemas for those with a robust constitution who were not eliminating properly; he recommended suppositories for those with a weak constitution. Other ancient Greek physicians, such as Galen in the second century A.D., utilized enemas in their practice as well.

Chang Chung Ching, whom some call the "Chinese Hippocrates," used enemas and allegedly preferred them to cathartic herbs.[8] Cathartic herbs are those that strongly purge the bowels and usually have an irritating effect on the colon's walls.

Ayurvedic medicine, which developed in India and dates back as far as 5,000 years, is practiced in the U.S. today. Ayurveda utilizes a variety of enemas and colon cleanses administered according to body type, constitution, and disease syndrome.[9] Based on these criteria, many different substances were used in Ayurvedic enemas. For example, sesame oil was thought to provide lubrication to the colon wall. Such substances, however, have no lasting effect in normalizing the colon flora or restoring the slightly acid pH.

Regnier de Graaf was a prominent Dutch physician who lived from 1641 to 1673. He studied medicine in Holland, England, and France, specializing in research and anatomical study. He was the first to study pancreatic function and secretions and to recognize the importance of pancreatic juice in digestion. In 1672, he was the first to describe the structure of what we now call the Graafian follicles in the ovaries. In his medical practice, de Graaf used enemas and even created a syringe that patients could use at home for their ease and convenience. Up until this time, assistance was necessary for administration of enemas. He recommended enemas for many intestinal complaints and also found them effective for problems in the bladder, kidney, and uterus, and for relief of headaches.[10]

Today, enemas provide a simple way to relieve the colon at home. Colonics are usually performed by trained laypersons using special apparatus to gently flush water through the colon at extremely low pressure. Water colonics and enemas, while helpful to remove waste matter, are not complete in their approach. They are useful in alleviating symptoms but do not address the root cause. The missing piece of information is the scientific knowledge of the correct colon pH. Water enemas and colonics leave the colon in an alkaline condition, which will support the growth of putrefactive bacteria. Acidophilus is unable to grow in an alkaline colon.

Water is a neutral pH of 7.0. The action of water can sweep out beneficial bacteria, weakened by living in an alkaline pH, along with harmful bacteria. Oxygen colonics are considered useful for destroying parasites but also will destroy acidophilus, which can live only in an oxygen-free environment.[11] Implants and enemas done with herbs, wheat grass, or coffee may have some temporary beneficial effects but ultimately fail because they leave the colon in an alkaline condition, vulnerable to immediate proliferation of the harmful, putrefactive bacteria, yeast, fungi, and even parasites. Water colonics also deplete the system of electrolytes.

When the colon is in such an alkaline condition, it does not matter how many billions of acidophilus are introduced orally or rectally. They will rapidly die because no foundation for their growth has been laid. Before acidophilus can be introduced, the colon must first be reacidified naturally.

Human Acidophilus for Human Colons

Only a human strain of acidophilus will be able to implant in the human colon. Most strains on the store shelves today are of animal origin. If the colon flora is severely damaged, the colon must be cleansed and restored to its slightly acid pH before acidophilus can be implanted rectally. This is the only way to ensure effective and lasting results.

In 1899, Professor Metchnikoff applied what he called "replacement therapy" when he experimented with implanting *Lactobacillus bulgaricus*, a beneficial bacteria, in the colon to eliminate harmful disease-forming species. As we noted previously, ever since this first unsuccessful experiment, replacement therapy has been a major area of interest in the quest for colon health. Again, his therapy failed only because *L. bulgaricus* is a strain of acidophilus from cows that will not implant in a human colon.

In 1980, only five or six acidophilus products were available in health food stores. But by 1993, according to the retail industry's *Whole Food Source Book*, this figure jumped to 120 acidophilus products, not including those sold exclusively by health professionals.

In 1989, the National Nutritional Foods Association (NNFA) adopted a labeling standard for probiotics. However, this standard does not include identifying whether the source of the bacteria is human or animal, a most unfortunate oversight. Acidophilus must be of human origin to implant in a human colon. Strains of acidophilus from cows, other animals, birds, or plants will not take up residency and live in the human colon.[12] Each species has its own biochemistry and microecosystem requirements. Growth factors for acidophilus found in milk vary from species to species as well, because the bacterial strains differ.[13] Many acidophilus products on the market are of bovine (cow) origin. To find out if the source of your acidophilus product is human or animal, ask your retailer or call the company yourself. Ask them for scientific data to back up their claims.

A high-grade, strong acidophilus strain that is viable (alive) and contains a high count of live acidophilus is necessary. Since acidophilus are sensitive to light and oxygen, many products deteriorate rapidly and do not remain viable for long. If the count is not high enough, the implant will not be successful. The count should be at least 100 billion for a successful rectal implant. (Refer to Appendix B for more clarification here.)

Questions and Answers

Q. *How long after WIT™ does it take for the acidophilus to get established?*

A. Usually it takes 3 to 4 weeks for the acidophilus to become established and predominant in the colon. The stool is an indicator. A floating stool that is soft but well formed, brown in color, with no odor is an indicator of a healthy acidophilus flora in the colon. Once you have regular, odorless elimination, determine how much Pro-Flora™ Whey you need to stay regular. Everyone requires a different amount. Generally 3 tablespoons in water once a day is effective although some people do well using this amount only a few times a week.

TABLE 6.
Assessing Colon Treatments and Products

Whenever you hear about a certain product or therapy, ask the following questions:

- What effect will it have on the colon pH?

- What will it do to reacidify the colon?

- What effects will it have on the acidophilus colon flora?

- Will it survive the stomach acids, bile, and trypsin to reach the colon?

- Does it achieve lasting results in the colon?

- What data are there to substantiate the claims?

- Are the data based on human, in vivo, studies?

- What is the source of the lactobacteria?

Q. *What else can I do to improve my elimination?*

A. When sitting on the toilet, place the feet on a small, low stool so as to be in a semisquatting position, with the knees raised up. This relieves the strain on the colon and facilitates elimination as it is a more natural position.

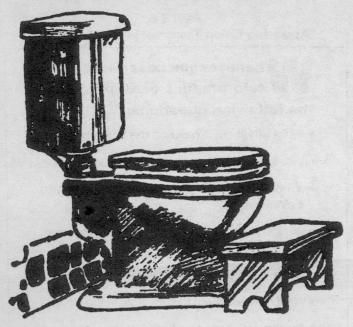

Figure 9. A Footstool by the Toilet Aids Elimination

Q. *I have been diagnosed with colitis by my doctor. Will your approach help me?*

A. Colitis is a major medical problem. Everyone with colitis is unique due to differences in his or her constitution, duration of the problem, and what medications he or she is taking and has taken in the past. Natural approaches may or may not be helpful depending on the individual. You need to consult with your physician for appropriate care. The colon has been at an alkaline pH for quite some time in order for a person to develop colitis.

My approach is primarily through prevention. However, with a doctor's supervision, this and other natural procedures may be implemented.

Q. *I have been diagnosed with colon cancer. Will colonics help me?*

A. Cancer is a medical problem that only a qualified physician may treat. Colonics are contraindicated in this condition. Colonics and the WIT™ procedure are for prevention only. Cancer requires medical treatment and you should see your physician.

Q. *I am three months pregnant and constipated. Will colonics be helpful for me?*

A. No. Colonics should not be done while pregnant. The best approach is prevention. The colon should be cleared and normalized before pregnancy.

Q. *Will wheat grass promote the growth of acidophilus?*

A. No. Wheat grass is alkaline and will not provide food for acidophilus whether taken orally or rectally. When taken orally, wheat grass is absorbed in the stomach and small intestine and will not reach the colon. When implanted rectally, it creates an alkaline pH in the colon favorable to the growth of harmful bacteria.

Q. *I've been using colon cleansers and laxatives to help my colon. Aren't these helpful to restore the colon flora?*

A. An old practice still popular among health practitioners and laypeople alike is the use of colon cleansers or laxatives to move the bowels. The average person today uses laxatives excessively to the detriment of his health. Although these laxative products are not intended for daily or long-term use, most of them are being used in just that manner.

Many herbal colon cleansers on the market contain senna, rhubarb, cascara sagrada, or other herbs that irritate the colon lining. These herbs are meant for only occasional use in extreme conditions. All colon cleansers provide only temporary symptomatic relief. The underlying cause of poor elimination, an incorrect colon pH, is not being addressed. Poor diet along with overuse of laxative products only makes the problem worse.

10

FEED YOUR ACIDOPHILUS WITH WHEY!

■

The fountain of youth is within! When the colon is out of balance, it is possible to restore the slightly acid pH and acidophilus flora which is our internal fountain of youth.

In over twenty years of experience and research, I have seen only two time-proven effective methods for restoring the acidophilus colon flora with lasting results. Both these approaches use edible-grade sweet dairy whey, which is the key factor to change the colon from alkaline to acid and to promote the growth of the acidophilus flora by providing the essential nutrients they require. Edible-grade, sweet dairy whey needs to be included in the daily diet to ensure long-term colon health.

When the acidophilus flora is depleted but some still remain, many people find they can restore their colon to health simply by drinking whey on a regular basis. They are able to monitor the status of their colon health by observing the regularity and quality of their bowel movements. Usually, these positive changes are observed within 4 to 8 weeks of drinking 1 to 3 tablespoons of whey in a glass of water daily.

Years ago, my neighbor was a professional landscape

gardener. One morning he came by to show me a check for three thousand dollars he had received to buy plants for a job. He said, "Before I take my crew in to plant these, I'm going to check the soil pH. If the soil pH isn't correct, the plants won't live long because they won't get proper assimilation of the nutrients they need to grow." He understood the natural laws of cause and effect and balance. The soil in the body is the colon acidophilus flora. We cannot keep breaking natural laws and expect to be healthy. Sweet edible dairy whey helps to correct the pH of the colon soil so the acidophilus flora can take root there, and also provides the nutrients required by acidophilus to grow.

Most people can transform their colon flora from a pathogenic to a protective flora by using sweet, edible whey orally as part of their daily diet. As far as the acidophilus flora is concerned, whey is the adult version of breast milk because it contains all the nutrients necessary for the multiplication of colon acidophilus.

As we have seen, a healthy diet and good digestion are essential for colon health. In addition, specific foods promote the growth of acidophilus. This is what we will now explore. Acidophilus have complex nutritional requirements similar to that of their human hosts. Their primary need is for carbohydrates. Lactose (milk sugar) is the specific food for acidophilus, which also require some amino acids, vitamins, minerals, and fatty acids. The food naturally highest in these nutrients in correct proportions for acidophilus proliferation is human-grade, sweet dairy whey. Acidophilus ferment the carbohydrate lactose. This process produces the beneficial acids that keep our colon healthy.

The pH of whey is about 6.0, which is slightly acid, making it ideal for maintenance of the digestive tract.

Whey acts as a natural antiseptic, destroying or inhibiting the growth of pathogenic microorganisms while causing no harm to human tissues.

Lactose: Food for Acidophilus

Lactose is the only common sugar that reaches the colon in large amounts and is the primary carbohydrate required by acidophilus bacteria. Lactose is one of the growth factors in mother's milk that promotes multiplication of the original *B. bifidum* implant in an infant's colon. The fact that lactose reaches the colon largely undigested makes complete sense when we realize its primary role is as food for acidophilus residing there. As always, nature has a plan.

Whole, sweet edible-grade whey is the food highest in naturally occurring lactose and is a natural, balanced food that contains all the nutrients required by acidophilus in appropriate proportions.[1] It consists of 60 percent lactose, 12 percent lactalbumin protein, and 11 percent minerals. Whey is the liquid essence of milk separated out during the cheese-making process and contains no fat or casein, as these go into the cheese. Whey contains anywhere from about 1 to 4 percent butter fat as compared with 25 to 40 percent in cheese. Since many people are allergic to casein or have trouble with the high fat content of most cheeses, people can often tolerate whey better than cheese or milk.

Studies show that the growth of colon acidophilus can be promoted by simply providing sufficient quantities of lactose. In a study done by the Food and Drug Administration (FDA), an initial dose of 240 to 400 grams of lactose was found to be effective in promoting colonization of the colon without any additional acidophilus being ingested.[2]

TABLE 7.
Conditions Favorable for Proliferation of Acidophilus[3]

No matter how many acidophilus are introduced into the colon, if the conditions are not favorable, they will rapidly die. The following conditions are favorable to their growth:

- Anaerobiosis
- A pH value between 5.0 and 7.0
- A fermentable sugar or other source of energy
- An assimilable source of nitrogen (*e.g.*, a protein hydrolysate)
- Necessary growth factors
- Necessary minerals and trace elements

Other factors in the colon that may affect growth are:
- Surface tension
- Presence of antibiotics or other substances

Notes:
- Given the conditions listed above, acidophilus can ferment sugars (most notably lactose) to produce acid and create the environment favorable for themselves in the colon.

- The only common sugars that can pass through the stomach into the colon in any quantity are lactose and dextrin.

Many people see beneficial changes in their elimination and colon health simply by including whey in their daily diet.

Whey: An Ancient Remedy

In Sweden, whey cheese and whey butter were once made and consumed daily. Sweet dairy whey can be used on oatmeal, cereals, as a beverage, or in blended drinks. It can be used as a substitute for milk products in baking and cooking with delicious results. Historically, Hippocrates, the Father of Medicine, suggested whey for the health of his patients. The diary of Samuel Pepys, a seventeenth-century admiral in the English Navy, is most intersting in this regard. Pepys wrote about frequenting places where whey was served regularly. He said, "Thence to the whey house and drank a great deal of whey and so home." The story of Little Miss Muffet eating her curds and whey is said to have originated in Scandinavia. Here they drank whey for centuries as it was known for its health benefits and thought to be the secret of their beautiful complexions. The noted Dr. Paavo Airola called whey a "miracle food" to help people stay young and healthy longer. Whey is the liquid gold essence of milk that supports our immune system and maintains our protective flora throughout life. This long-forgotten, valuable food should again be made part of our regular diet for good colon health.

Whey Protein

The amino acids in whey have about 98 percent bioavailability and contain all the essential amino acids in excess of the requirements of the reference protein of the World

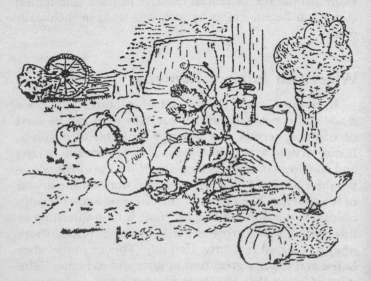

Figure 10. Little Miss Muffet

Health Organization.[4] Research shows whey protein to be superior to soy, rice, wheat, or beef as far as quality and bioavailability. The soluble protein lactoglobulins in whey are identical to serum globulin found in human blood and contain antibodies that help strengthen the immune system.[5] The major soluble proteins in whey are beta-lactoglobulin, immunoglobulin, alpha-lactalbumin, and serum albumin.[6] Today, whey protein isolates are very popular among athletes in-training due to the high bioavailability and excellent amino acid profile.

Whey Protein Isolates

Whey protein powders that have been processed by methods that do not denature the amino acids are found to enhance immune function. Many whey protein powders have been hydrolyzed which uses enzymes to break the amide bonds within the proteins, so they'll be smaller and easier to assimilate. They provide amino acid precursors to the important antioxidant glutathione which plays multiple roles in our bodies. Glutathione supports lymphocyte function, acts as an antioxidant, regulates other antioxidants, and acts as a detoxifying agent at the cellular level.

Of course, whey protein powders are isolates. The amino acid component of whey has been extracted and the lactose has been removed. Therefore whey protein isolates are not complete foods, and since they contain little or no lactose, they will not stimulate growth of the natural colon flora. They are incomplete because they do not contain lactose or the complete nutritional profile contained in whole whey that is required by the acidophilus bacteria. Whey protein isolate powder can be mixed with whole, sweet, edible-grade whey to get the benefits of both. Taken together, a whey protein isolate that benefits the immune system, combined with whole, sweet dairy whey that feeds the acidophilus, is a terrific boost for the whole body.

Edible-Grade Whey

There are basically two different grades of whey available on the market today. The most commonly found type of whey is standard-grade whey which has been marketed for human use. Usually the taste of this whey is marginal to sour or salty and it does not mix well in water. When I

TABLE 8.
Comparison of Whey Protein Quality
and Bioavailability[7,8,9]

Protein	Chemical Score	Biological Value*	Net Protein Value**
Whey	>100	104	92
Egg	100	94	94
Fish	71	76	80
Beef	69	74	67
Casein	58	80	72
Oats	57	65	66
Rice	56	64	57
Soybeans	47	73	61
Wheat	43	65	40
Lentils	31	45	30

*Biological Value shows the actual protein use in adults.
**Net Protein Value shows the amount of protein assimilable by adults.

first began this work, I found little or no compliance with my recommendation that everyone drink whey regularly. People did not like the taste of whey and found it difficult to mix and use easily. Now I find tremendous compliance and excellent results using an edible-grade whey that has been specially prepared for human consumption, is deliciously sweet, and mixes well in water. (Refer to Appendix B for more clarification here.) According to the grading system used by the United States Department of Agriculture, the classification of "Edible Grade Whey" is given to identify whey made especially for human consumption. So many people tell me their stories of how they have benefited from using this sweet, edible-grade whey. couple reported the quality of their sleep each night improved and they both had more energy during the day. Many people who have suffered from irregularity, constipation, and even diarrhea report normalization of their colon just from using edible sweet whey. Gas pains, bad odor, and intestinal discomfort are often relieved just through use of whey within seven to thirty days. Whey should be a continual part of the diet to keep the internal environment clean and keep the colon in a healthy condition, free of toxin-forming bacteria.

A dog lover told me he even gave a tablespoon of whey to his golden retriever in his daily food because his veterinarian recommended he do so. His dog was very regular with no bad odors.

A woman had upper and lower gastrointestinal examinations. The doctors found nothing physically wrong and diagnosed her with irritable bowel syndrome. After a week of using sweet, edible-grade whey, she reported her elimination became regular again and has remained so ever since.

Another woman wrote, "I consider myself to be in good health. I keep an eye on what I eat, try to minimize fats and sugar in my diet, and drink only about one glass of red wine a week. I exercise regularly. Since I started drinking sweet dairy whey, I notice an improvement in what I already considered a happy lifestyle. My lower back feels better and the occasional back spasms have diminished. The main difference is in my 'plumbing.' I am very regular and consistent. I also honestly feel a lot more energetic."

A 78-year-old woman complained of constipation most of her life. After drinking the whey I recommended for almost four weeks, she almost completely stopped taking the herbal laxatives she had depended on for years. She

she then went in for an exam, her ___ ___ old her that her colon was unusually ___ ___ looking.

___ ___ ___ceived a letter from an 84-year-old woman who kne___ ___ Empringham. She wrote, "It was my great good fortune to meet up with Dr. Empringham in about 1934 when I was 20. We had little knowledge of food and health in those depression years and symptoms of colitis appeared. Luckily, at this time, I read in a health article that Dr. Empringham was here from England and would be giving colonics. I went to him for three colonics in one week and he reimplanted my colon with human lactobacillus. My troubles were over and I am eternally grateful to him!"

Another woman recently wrote me, "Thank you for getting me to use the whey! After years of constipation problems, even before the constipating antibiotics, everything is getting back to normal."

Transforming the Acidophilus Colon Flora Orally

Start with 1 tablespoon of sweet edible whey added to 1 cup purified water. After 2 or 3 days, slowly increase the amount to 3 tablespoons. If you are not getting results, then increase the amount of whey to up to 6 tablespoons a day. If any gas or discomfort is felt, discontinue the whey for a day.

While you are first using the whey orally to try to boost your natural acidophilus flora, abstain from gas-forming foods, alcohol, beans, broccoli, and any other foods that cause you digestive discomfort. Also cut down on any flesh foods, especially red meats, that can cause putrefaction and delay establishment of the beneficial flora.

Whey Recipes
YOGURT SHAKE

5 tablespoons natural yogurt (Refer to Appendix B.)
1 cup filtered water or organic milk (Refer to Appendix B.)
1 to 2 tablespoons of sweet whey
1 teaspoon to 1 tablespoon organic raw honey to taste
Fresh, organic fruit to taste. (Do not use acid fruits such
*   as oranges. Use fruits such as apples, berries, or*
*   papayas.)*

Combine all ingredients in a blender and blend to the consistency of a milkshake.

DAVE'S SUPER ENERGY SMOOTHIE

1 ripe banana
3 tablespoons whole, sweet, edible-grade whey (Refer to
*   Appendix B.)*
1 teaspoon green drink (Refer to Appendix B.)
2 cups organic milk or filtered water (Refer to Appendix
*   B.)*
2 drops vanilla
1 teaspoon to 1 tablespoon of organic raw honey
½ cup cooked rice cereal (See recipe in Chapter 12.)

Combine all ingredients in a blender and blend until smooth.

Breakfast Cereal for You and Your Acidophilus

Mix 2 to 3 tablespoons of sweet dairy whey in a glass of filtered water. Just before eating, pour whey drink over your fresh-ground, hot breakfast cereal.

If you like, add a pinch of cinnamon and a little honey or maple syrup.

Questions and Answers

Q. *I am lactose intolerant although I can eat yogurt. Will I be able to digest whey?*

A. Some people find they are lactose intolerant. There are several possible reasons for this. Some people are deficient in the lactose-digesting enzyme, lactase. Some people totally lack the enzyme. Many of these people, however, are able to digest fermented milk products. Some people who thought they were lactose intolerant report that, when their acidophilus colon flora is reestablished, they are able to digest lactose products that they were unable to digest previously. If you are able to digest yogurt, then usually you will be able to digest whey. Some people are not lactose intolerant but are intolerant to the casein protein found in dairy products. Lactose intolerance may be genetic, or may be caused by a deficiency of acidophilus in the colon, which leads to insufficient production of the enzyme lactase. In these cases, edible-grade, sweet whole whey feeds and stimulates the growth of acidophilus flora. (Refer to Appendix B for more clarification here.)

If you think you are lactose intolerant, you can start with as little as 1 teaspoon of whey. Gradually increase the

amount to 1 to 3 tablespoons. Some people (
sweet whey mixed in warm foods or drinks.

Q. *How much sweet edible whey should I use?*

A. Whey is a natural and safe food that may be consumed freely. To feed your acidophilus, a minimum of 3 to 4 tablespoons mixed in water and included regularly in the daily diet will be most effective. You can determine for yourself the optimum amount and frequency of using whey by monitoring your stools as described in this book and adjusting the amount of whey so they reflect the presence of a healthy acidophilus colon flora.

Q. *Can children use sweet edible-grade whey?*

A. Many mothers report excellent results with their children, especially when they were breastfed and have a foundation of good flora. One woman told me her 6-year-old had diarrhea for some time. After she gave her as little as 1 teaspoon of whey on her cereal each morning, her stools became normal. Usually for children weighing up to 50 pounds, 1 teaspoon of sweet whey is sufficient. For best flavor and consistency, usually 1 to 3 tablespoons in a glass of filtered water is a general guideline.

Q. *Since whey is such a wonderful food and promotes the growth of acidophilus, can I feed it to my baby as formula? I am not able to breastfeed her.*

A. Absolutely nothing should be used as formula for infants without the consent of your family physician. Infant formulas are scientifically designed to meet all the infant's needs. Whey is known to be safe for children who are weaned and eating regular foods.

Q. *I have been told not to eat any type of sugars, natural or otherwise, because of* Candida. *How can I feed acidophilus in my colon without making* Candida *worse? Will the lactose (milk sugar) in whey feed the* Candida?

A. There is no evidence that lactose feeds *Candida*.[10] Most people can use whey orally with no problems at all. Those who cannot are able to feed the acidophilus directly by using a whey solution rectally to bypass the digestive tract. Four tablespoons of whey in one quart of water used as an enema once a week can stimulate the growth of acidophilus and help restore the natural bacterial balance.

Once *Candida* is eliminated, the colon should immediately be restored to its slightly acidic pH and reimplanted with acidophilus. Whey can then usually be tolerated and used to continue to feed acidophilus to help prevent recurrence of *Candida*. After 4 to 6 weeks a person may be able to tolerate whey orally. Try small amounts of whey at first and increase use slowly. You can start with only 1 teaspoon of whey a day. If this is agreeable, slowly increase the amount daily up to 3 tablespoons per day. When you have a condition such as *Candida*, it is always advisable to consult with your physician before trying something new.

Q. *I have been on different cleansing programs over the years. I have tried psyllium, bentonite, liver flushes, lots of herbal colon cleansers, wheat grass enemas, and a yeast-free diet with no sugar or breads. I am still constipated and experience terrible-smelling gas and bloating that gets worse when I eat certain things. Is there anything I can do?*

A. Even if your colon had an acid pH when you first began these programs, it is apparent from your complaints that your colon is now in an alkaline condition. I would suggest starting simply. Eat soft, cooked foods such as complex carbohydrates and vegetables as described in this book. Include soups in your regular diet and drink enough purified, clean water. The moisture will help move out the hard stool. Eat some salads, but use flesh foods sparingly. Eggs are preferable as a protein source during the transition period. Make sure they are fertile eggs from range-fed chickens for optimal nutrition. Gradually add liquid whey into your diet, which will begin to normalize your colon pH and supply nutrients for any latent acidophilus there. Follow the program outlined in this book. Be relaxed when you eat and allow quiet time for digestion after meals.

Q. *You mentioned other carbohydrates, such as dextrin, that can be utilized by the acidophilus colon flora. Please explain more.*

A. Maltose and dextrin are secondary carbohydrates that can be utilized by the acidophilus. Maltose is found in malt, which is germinated from whole barley. Dextrin is formed in the digestive tract as a result of digesting complex carbohydrates, including whole grains. A study done by the FDA found dextrin also to be effective in colonizing the intestine without the use of oral lactobacteria.[11] This is one reason why a diet high in natural whole grains and complex carbohydrates is so beneficial to colon health that we include a chapter on whole grains.

Lactose in whey exerts the strongest dietary influence in transforming the colon flora to one predominated by acidophilus because it supplies all their nutritional needs for growth. Maltose and dextrin, from digestion of complex carbohydrates, are important secondary foods that assist in promoting a strong, positive influence on the beneficial acidophilus colon flora.[12]

Q. *I have been using whey protein for 6 months as I have read that it is high in amino acids. I still have a lot of gas. What is going on?*

A. I have been asked this question many times since whey protein products have been on the market. Whey protein powder supplies excellent-quality clean protein that replenishes the cell. However, whey protein is an isolate of whey, not a whole food product—it contains only the protein aspect of whey. Whey protein does not contain lactose, which is the essential factor to promote acidophilus growth, along with the other minerals and nutrients required by acidophilus. Whole sweet dairy whey contains all the nutrients necessary to feed and multiply acidophilus in the colon and in so doing can eliminate gas-forming bacteria, which will live only in an alkaline pH.

11

NUTRITION, LIFESTYLE, AND COLON HEALTH

■

Nature did not intend nutrition to be confusing, yet many people are so confused they have lost the basic knowledge of what to eat! I see many people who are experiencing toxicity not only from an unhealthy colon, but also from consuming an excess of the wrong foods or poor digestion. Poorly digested food enters the colon and contributes to stagnation and formation of an alkaline pH. Eventually, the combination of a toxic colon and deficient diet culminates in illness and fatigue. Reaching this point, people think they need some sort of supplement or herb in order to resolve their various ailments. Taking a shotgun approach, they overwhelm the system, consuming multitudes of natural and synthetic supplements from their ever-expanding home pharmacy, hoping something will hit the right place and all will be well again.

But they are still sick and tired. The shotgun approach is similar to flooding the carburetor in a car. The body is unable to metabolize supplements taken in excess. Too much is as bad as too little. We need to take a step back and assess the person's status.

First, you must normalize the colon; then follow a balanced diet and lifestyle for lasting results. This is the foundation. It is a foundation that will enable you to take care of remaining health concerns appropriately and successfully.

Factors to consider when planning a diet are one's constitution, present state of health, quality and quantity of foods, the current amount of physical and mental activity, climate, environment, and stress level. Become aware of the effects and ease of digestion of foods. Find foods that impart energy and a sense of well-being, and enable you to achieve your goals in life. Moderation is the key. Many people become depleted simply from years of food fanaticism and continual cleansing diets. When the body is strong, healthy, nourished properly, and with a healthy colon, it will clean itself without any radical efforts. Provide adequate nourishment by including generous helpings of fresh, cooked vegetables and whole grains as the basis of your diet.

Whole Foods, Balanced Diet

A whole food diet of high-quality foods ensures the best-quality nutrients. Much more than just so many units of nutrients or calories, food imparts life force or vitality to us. Only fresh food can impart this quality of life force or living energy. Modern science realizes that nutrients and enzymes are more abundant in fresh foods than in old foods. Storage, manufacturing, or shipping procedures compromise the nutrient capacity and life force present in foods.

We were not meant to live on a diet consisting of canned, processed, and frozen foods. Such foods may contain nutrients but have little or no life force or enzymes. They should constitute only a very small part, if any, of your diet.

Digestion is the first step in overall good health. If you digest your food well, you support your body nutritionally with the building and repair blocks necessary for daily life. Then and only then can you support yourself emotionally, mentally, and spiritually with the fuel to carry out necessary activities.

Most aware health professionals today recommend a balanced diet of 70 to 80 percent complex carbohydrates (including grains, vegetables, and fruits), 15 percent protein, and about 15 percent natural fats. Studies show this dietary balance promotes health and also encourages the growth and maintenance of acidophilus in the colon.[1,2]

Studies show that in countries with low fat and protein intake, combined with high-fiber consumption in the form of complex carbohydrates, grains, and vegetables, there is a very low incidence of colon and other health problems.[3,4] In our modern society, nutritionists are now finding many problems due to the high-carbohydrate diet many people are on, with very low amounts of protein and fats. There needs to be a balance. Remember: All the cell walls of the body are composed of proteins and fats, which are absolutely necessary for cellular repair and proper physical functioning.

Carbohydrates

Complex carbohydrates are a primary source of energy for the body and along with vegetables provide the best source of natural fiber for the system. Since acidophilus thrive on a high percentage of complex carbohydrates, this also serves as a guideline for consideration.

Complex carbohydrates include potatoes, sweet potatoes, squash, pumpkin, brown rice and other whole grains.

Generous servings of vegetables at lunch and dinner are excellent. Many vegetables, herbs, and fruits can be organically grown in the backyard, with very little investment of time and money. For the busy person, many health food stores carry a selection of fresh, organic produce. The organic food industry is growing by leaps and bounds as the public becomes aware of the dangers of pesticide contamination. Pesticides can overload the liver and the body tissues with toxins. The extra time and price in choosing and paying for organic foods is worth its weight in gold! Avoiding pesticide contamination found in produce and eating thoughtfully and organically is your safest ticket to health.

Protein

Protein needs vary from person to person. Many Americans today consume a diet of about 40% fats/oils, 40% refined sugars, and about three times the recommended daily allowance of protein. The necessary amount of protein in the diet is a subject of constant controversy. Protein is essential for maintenance, repair, and growth of the body. Unless you are physically active, however, protein intake can all too easily become excessive.

Foods high in protein are necessary for some individuals, especially when they exert substantial physical, mental, or emotional energy. Most people do not do well in the long term on a vegetarian diet. Those who do are fortunate because most animals today are not raised under ideal conditions, leading to poor-quality animal food products. Cattle may be eating pesticide-sprayed grass and feed. Animals are fed hormones to increase their growth rate and are given antibiotics to fend off the incidence of disease.

Due to the prevalence of polluted water, many fish contain chemicals and heavy metals. The larger the body of the fish, the greater the accumulation of contaminants. One of the culprits in the current overuse of antibiotics discussed earlier is their widespread occurrence in our diets, owing to their use in raising livestock and fish. In meat products and commercially raised fish, even trace amounts of antibiotics build up in humans when such foods are consumed daily and in combination.

Many health food stores carry natural, range-fed, hormone-free animal products that have been raised without antibiotics. If you are one of the people who needs occasional animal protein, this is your best option to provide yourself with excellent quality.

Fats and Oils

Fats and oils are essential for all body functions, lubrication, brain function, and hormonal production. They are also important in the immune system and to modulate inflammatory and healing responses in the body. The kinds of oils we eat influence all these areas of our health. Avoid all hydrogenated or partially hydrogenated oils, which are not healthy. Read product labels because many products contain these harmful hydrogenated fats. Margarine and shortening are hydrogenated and should be avoided as well. Use natural, time-proven oils or organic butter for your health. The best-quality oils are those found in health food stores, as they have been processed without the use of harsh, toxic chemicals and are usually expelled at lower temperatures to preserve their nutrient value. (Refer to Appendix B for more clarification here.)

Undoubtedly, olive oil is best for cooking and salad

dressing. This time-proven oil is high in nutrients and very beneficial to the body. Olive oil also stores well and can withstand cooking temperatures. Sesame oil is another stable, nutritious, and flavorful oil that can be used in cooking.

Omega-3 oils are now becoming well known for their role in immunity, brain function, and overall health. Include fish such as salmon and rainbow trout in your diet as excellent sources of both omega-3 oils and protein. Liquid, refrigerated flax oil or flax with borage oil is also excellent nutritional support in getting omega-3 fatty acids on a regular basis. (Refer to Appendix B for more clarification here.)

Digestion

It's not only what we eat that's important, but what we digest and assimilate. If food is not digested properly, it will arrive at the colon undigested and this can lead to colon problems.

If food is not being digested properly, people will experience symptoms such as bloating, discomfort, gas or belching after eating, constipation or diarrhea, bad breath, and inappropriate weight loss or gain. Undigested food noticed in the stools is a clear sign of poor digestion. The first key to good digestion is to eat healthful foods and find those that suit your body type, climate, and lifestyle.

Otherwise, there are a variety of digestive enzymes to choose from to help your digestion on a daily basis. I prefer plant-derived enzymes that contain amylase, protease, lipase, and cellulase. Amylase assists carbohydrate digestion, protease assists protein digestion, and lipase improves digestion of fats. Cellulase specifically helps digestion of the fibrous matter in vegetables and fruits. Even though small quantities of enzymes do exist in foods, a small amount of supplementary plant-derived enzymes is an easy way to boost our own digestive powers. Edward Howell, Ph.D., biochemist and nutrition researcher, was the first to recognize and describe the role of food enzymes in human nutrition. He developed enzymes that would compensate for the deficiencies in the human food chain. Dr. Howell's book, *Enzyme Nutrition,* is the culmination of 20 years of study. It is the short version of his original 700-page book, which contained over 700 scientific references.[5] I recommend it highly.

Warm Foods for Warm Bodies

When we eat, our bodies warm the food to body temperature in order to digest it. That is one reason why too many cold, raw foods deplete our digestive functioning. Many individuals experience indigestion and gas from eating raw foods. Most people do best with about 80 to 90 percent cooked foods and 10 to 20 percent raw vegetables and fruits. This varies seasonally and according to the person. In the cold of winter, anyone with common sense will eat very few, if any, raw, cold foods. Warm foods help nourish us at all levels to keep us warm, happy people in warm, healthy bodies.

Cooking makes many nutrients available for assimilation by the body, such as the B vitamins in string beans. Gently steaming vegetables with small amounts of water conserves the most nutrients and keeps the most natural taste.

Eating uncooked grains, no matter how long they are soaked, places a great strain on the digestive tract and can cause congestion in the colon. Cooked grains are digested well and provide the best nutrition.

Quality Water

Good, pure water is essential for all the cells and tissues in our bodies, and thus for our health. Unfortunately, hundreds of chemicals are now present in our drinking water.

The Environmental Protection Agency (EPA) claims that 800 water systems, serving 30 million people, have excessive levels of lead in their drinking water. The effects of lead in the human system include miscarriages, infants with low birth weight, and central nervous system disorders in the young. Adults are at risk for high blood pressure and kidney disease.[6] The presence of lead is only one example of the many problems associated with drinking water in America. In order to avoid consuming these chemicals and pesticides that leach into the water system, we must purify our water.

For providing pure drinking water, machine dispensers and bottled water are not as cost-effective as owning a home filter system. In recent years, many improved purification units have appeared on the market, so the consumer will need to do a little research before investing in a water purifier.

Many different types of units are available, but not all are effective in removing impurities. Any purification unit used should be tested by an independent source in order to confirm its effectiveness. Verify that the product has been tested and certified by the National Sanitation Foundation (NSF), which is one such foundation for independent testing and information.

A 0.5-micron pore size is necessary to filter out *Giardia lamblia* and *Cryptosporidium*, waterborne parasites that are found in many water supplies today and which can cause diarrhea, gas, intestinal discomfort, and other problems. Despite methods used in water purification plants, there have been many outbreaks of these organisms, outbreaks widely reported in *Newsweek*, *The Wall Street Journal*, and other publications throughout the past decade. In 1993, *Infectious Disease News* reported that 281,000 people in Milwaukee were infected by *Cryptosporidium* in the city's water supply.[7]

Some individuals find reverse-osmosis systems to produce satisfactory water. I prefer a solid carbon-block filter system that retains the naturally occurring minerals in water. Although distilled water is sometimes useful during a detoxification program, nature does not produce distilled water. We need the mineral components found in naturally clean water. Distillation will not remove pesticides from water either. A good solid-carbon block filtration system attached to your kitchen sink will remove pesticides, bacteria, and heavy metals. (Refer to Appendix A for more clarification here.)

Yogurt

A book on colon health would not be complete without mentioning yogurt, an ancient food that has been used by nomadic tribes around the world. The tribes made yogurt by transforming the milk of their herds with live starter cultures of bacteria. Children were breastfed and the constant use of yogurt helped maintain their colon flora for life. Yogurt starter cultures were prized, passed down from generation to generation, and shared among families. The source of their starter culture was, and still is, either from cows, sheep, camels, or horses. The cultures were live and very strong. Today's commercial yogurt is very weak by comparison and many of the cultures used are not ideal. Bovine-source lactobacteria are used commercially to transform milk into yogurt and most companies pasteurize the yogurt after the culture has been added, which kills the bacterial culture.

For the best-quality yogurt, look for brands that use *Lactobacillus acidophilus* and *Bifidobacterium bifidum.* The label should specifically state that the cultures were added after pasteurization. This type of yogurt will help maintain the colon flora, especially with the addition of an edible-grade, sweet whey.

Acidophilus milk and yogurt are popular, nutritious, and delicious foods. They will not, however, transform the colon flora into a beneficial flora for many of the same reasons discussed in earlier chapters. Studies show that both yogurt and acidophilus milk are useful health products, but you should not count on them to replenish a depleted colon flora.

Food Follies

People constantly ask me what foods will help or harm their colon flora. Occasionally, after a session, people call to complain about gas or digestive discomfort. Each time, after I question them, the cause has been one of the foods in this chapter. One woman went home and ate only a bagel for lunch, but couldn't understand why she had so much gas and discomfort. When the colon has been emptied and the beneficial flora is being reestablished, it is important to eat nutritious, cooked foods that digest easily for at least 5 or 6 days until the colon refills.

The foods discussed below are those that, from my experience, cause the most colon problems. There may be other foods that cause problems for an individual, according to his or her constitution or tolerance. Certain foods will actually cause or contribute to long- or short-term colon problems. There are also foods that will cause problems for some people and not others. The foods I am presenting here, across the board, are harmful to the acidophilus colon flora. You need to determine for yourself which foods are helpful and which foods are not.

Gas-Forming Foods

Very often, raw vegetables cause intestinal gas in people. Broccoli, cabbage, and cauliflower are particular problems for many individuals. Steam your vegetables or sauté them lightly in olive oil to get the best nutritional value, preserve valuable enzymes, and improve digestibility and bio-availability of nutrients.

The most common complaint from people is that eating beans gives them gas. This indicates that the beans are probably not being digested correctly. As a result, they end up in the colon undigested and cause gas. Use common sense. If any food gives you gas, don't eat it. If a food doesn't agree with you, you will not assimilate it properly.

Some people find they can tolerate beans if they sprout their beans for two to three days before cooking them. Cover your beans with water. Let them stand overnight. In the morning, drain off the soak water and add fresh water. Repeat the soak that evening and the following day. On the second or third day your beans will be starting to sprout and are ready to cook. The soaking and sprouting process helps remove the gas-forming component of the beans.

Dry Foods and Fiber

All dry foods tend to clog the colon and cause a variety of problems. These foods include bread, bagels, granola, bran products, and dried fruit. Include here as well powdered foods eaten with either insufficient or no liquids added, such as green algae tablets or powders, dry fiber bars, and the like.

Dehydrated food has had the water removed from it for convenient storage and extension of shelf life. Foods are not meant to be eaten in this form. They must be rehydrated before eating. This means, simply, that dried fruits can be softened in water overnight. Dry nutritional or algae powders should always be reconstituted in water before they are ingested.

When we eat foods that lack sufficient water content, our own body fluids will have to compensate for the deficiency. Excess consumption of dry, hard foods is a major cause of constipation.

Too much bread tends to keep the colon contents hard and dry. Many people do not digest bread well. Bagels cause gas and constipation in a large number of people. You will not crave bread if you increase your intake of freshly ground, cooked grains.

Popcorn is the king of dry foods. Its reputation as being a good source of fiber is a myth. Perhaps eating popcorn in moderation can be tolerated, but I have seen popcorn eaters who have terrible blockages in their colons. The outer husk of the popcorn kernel (the pieces that get caught in the teeth) is indigestible, hard, heat-treated cellulose. As an alternative to eating popcorn, I recommend a tasty rice product that is found in health food stores. Although the product looks and tastes like popcorn, it is completely free of kernels.

Fiber is an essential part of the diet, best consumed in its natural form, as found in fruits and vegetables, which have a high water content. Fiber products, isolated from whole foods, cause more problems than they solve. Combining incorrect types of fiber with a deficient colon flora interferes with normal elimination and actually makes for worse elimination problems. Get fiber in the forms made by nature: fresh fruits, vegetables, and cooked whole grains.

Alcohol

My clients often inquire about the effect of alcohol on their colon flora. I can only emphasize the point that alcohol must be used in moderation. Alcohol destroys the colon acidophilus. When clients drink any kind of alcohol, especially after implanting the acidophilus and during its period of reestablishment, the implant fails. To achieve a balanced immune system, forget alcohol instead of forgetting your health.

High-Protein, High-Fat Diets

Research shows that the main contributors to colon cancer around the world are diets high in fat and diets high in protein. Populations eating diets high in whole grains and vegetables and low in protein and fats have a low incidence of colon cancer, diabetes, and heart disease. These conditions rapidly increase with industrialization and are most prevalent in developed Western nations. The studies also show that high-protein diets combined with high fat intake cause harmful bacteria to proliferate in the colon and create toxic by-products.[8,9,10,11] When an excess of fats or oils is consumed, a flora is developed that can produce estrogens from the excess bile acids present in the colon. These estrogens can circulate in the bloodstream and contribute to many health problems.[12]

All animal proteins (including eggs) consumed in excess, without a balance of foods to stimulate acidophilus, lead to overgrowth of gas-forming proteolytic types of bacteria. This is accompanied by a corresponding decrease in acidophilus and a change in stool pH to alkaline.[13,14] In particular, too much red meat causes problems. Animal products are best consumed in moderation. Eating meat daily is eating meat too often. Red meats should be eaten only occasionally and in small amounts. Fish, fowl, and eggs are excellent sources of animal protein if they are raised naturally, without hormones and antibiotics.

Everyone today is concerned about fat. The problem is both the type and quantity of fats we are eating. Steam or gently stir-fry foods instead of deep frying. Use high-quality oils, such as olive or sesame, that have been cold-pressed without the use of heat or chemicals.[15,16,17]

Raw Protein Foods

Consuming raw fish from any location is really asking for trouble. Without a microscope, we are unable to see the parasites residing in raw fish and are unaware of their presence. Since these parasites are destroyed at normal cooking temperatures, the solution seems obvious. Cook your fish!

Some people eat raw eggs regularly. Many of them get *Salmonella* poisoning. The Centers for Disease Control report salmonellosis is increasing.

As the hazards from consuming raw dairy products

today are high, use only pasteurized milk.
ized society, where we do not personally o
hygiene, infection from a multiresistant or
Salmonella) increases. The possible risk   ...enefits
should be considered before eating any raw food.

Remedy for Problem Foods

One alternative is to include plant digestive enzymes
with your meal to see if digestion improves. If this eliminates the gas, you're fine. Otherwise, the answer is simply
to stop eating foods that constantly cause gas and other
digestive problems.

Find something else to eat. If you have gas for a few
days or longer, you need to take some steps to replenish the
good flora which have been challenged by the onslaught of
undigested food decomposing ungraciously in the colon.
In this case, increase the amount of sweet dairy whey to 2
or 3 glasses a day for several days. Usually, this eliminates
any gas and restores the healthy colon flora.

Enjoy Life!

Consider the foods you eat. Be aware of their effect on
you, your energy level, your moods, and your feeling of
well-being. Notice which foods are digested easily. Do you
feel satisfied after eating? Experiment with new foods. Find
and eat foods you enjoy, that impart sustained energy and
a sense of well-being, and that enable you to achieve your
goals in life.

You should not have to spend much time thinking
about your diet. Once you're in good health, with your
body in balance, it is easier to recognize both your basic
and changing needs. Your cravings will become healthier.

will want to move and exercise. Being in balance allows us to live our life with awareness of how to fulfill our needs simply in a harmonious way. You need to listen to yourself. Experiment; find out what works for you. Once you are on the right track, forget about your diet and enjoy life!

Questions and Answers

Q. *I never feel satisfied no matter how much I eat and I can't gain weight. Is this related to my colon health?*

A. These symptoms may be due to digestive enzyme imbalance, an alkaline colon, or to parasites. Plant digestive enzymes are available from most health food stores and help break down food, so it reaches the colon well digested. The difference in the stool is noticeable. If your food is not digesting well, particles of undigested food can often be seen in the stool. This will be alleviated after taking plant enzymes with meals. Microscopic parasites and/or worms can be ingested easily from raw fish, poorly cooked meat, unwashed vegetables, or improper hygiene. With the expansion of travel, parasites are also traveling and spreading around the planet. The presence of worms or parasites can cause either weight loss or obesity by taking nutrients from the system. They thrive in an alkaline pH. Your health professional can test for parasites. Do not self-treat for parasites. Always confirm their presence with laboratory tests.

12

GOLDEN GRAINS

■

Grains are truly the "staff of life" if they are prepared properly. Prior to industrialization, grains were hand ground with mortar and pestle immediately before cooking. This is still the practice in some areas of the world today, and we often see Third World women on television grinding grains in this manner. Close by is a pot of water in which the fresh, unoxidized grains will be cooked for a wholesome meal. In Chinese medicine, the word "chi" is loosely translated as "energy" or "life force." The Chinese character for chi includes the central image of steam rising up from a bowl of cereal grains. The body requires large amounts of complex carbohydrates in the form of grains and starchy vegetables to consistently provide us with the lasting energy we need on a daily and long-term basis.

Not All Carbohydrates Are Created Equal

We eat simple sugars, such as doughnuts, sugary candies, and cakes, for snacks and energy boosts. Metabolized quickly in the body, they often prompt a quick rise in blood sugar level, followed by a drop that leads to feelings of hypoglycemia, hunger, fatigue, or other symptoms as adrenaline takes over.

One of our problems with refined sugar and carbohydrates, such as candy, white sugar, and white flour products, concerns the large amount of glucose released into the body at once. In fact, the problem here is manifold. First, refined sugar and flour products have no nutritional value and, in fact, deplete the body of nutrition in the process of their absorption. This happens because the sharp rise and fall in blood sugar places stress on the adrenals and pancreas, which weakens the system. Further, there are not sufficient quantities of glucose to be stored up for later use. It is the same as when we are working incredibly hard at a stressful job, just living paycheck to paycheck with little or no money in savings.

To enhance glycogen stores in the body, we must first provide ourselves with fresh, high-quality complex carbohydrates such as whole grains, squashes, pumpkins and potatoes. These carbohydrates are released into the system more evenly and slowly over time, supplying a steady drip of nutrients into the system. When the blood sugar rises and falls rapidly, the body goes on red alert to correct these extremes. Fortunately, eating a good supply of freshly prepared complex carbohydrates is like working at a pleasant job and being able to put some money in the bank regularly. This allows you to build up reserves for present and future use. When the liver has a good glycogen reserve, we receive a steady glucose drip into the system and no longer crave candy bars, for instance, for a quick pick-me-up. Blood sugar stabilizes, and along with adequate protein intake and supplemental nutrition, low blood sugar problems are easily resolved.

When grains are ground and packaged, however, many essential nutrients are lost and the natural oils oxidize and become rancid. The body needs an adequate glycogen store in the liver which can best be supplied by consuming fresh ground, unoxidized grains. In the body, complex carbohydrates are broken down into glucose. Ideally, there is an excess of glucose, which the body stores in the liver as glycogen. When the need for energy arises, the body can rely on this store of glycogen and convert it to the glucose needed for physical activity, thinking, and other metabolic functions.

Whole, Freshly Ground Grains for Health

Grains should be purchased in their whole-seed form, with only the outer hull removed. They should be kept refrigerated until used to prevent spoilage. Grains can be cooked whole or ground in a grain mill prior to cooking. An electric blender or coffee grinder can also be used to grind grains. The advantages to using whole grains and grinding them freshly yourself are fivefold:

1. Nutrients are preserved well in fresh, whole grains.
2. Grinding grains fresh releases their nutrients, which are slightly broken down and therefore made more bioavailable just prior to cooking.
3. Cooking is the most nutrient-efficient way to prepare grains.
4. Ground grains cook quickly, usually in about 15 minutes.
5. They are delicious and can be prepared in a variety of ways.

Freshly ground grains cooked in this way are excellent as a breakfast cereal. You will notice more sustained energy throughout the day, and over time your overall energy level and performance will be higher. You will not feel hungry a half hour after breakfast. Freshly ground flour adds a wonderful array of flavor and nutrition to any of your cake, cookie, and bread recipes. Grains that can be used include hulled oats, rye, red winter wheat, spelt, millet, amaranth, quinoa, kamut, wild rice, or brown rice. Some people are gluten intolerant and may have trouble with grains high in gluten such as wheat, oats, or rye. If you suspect this, your doctor can use a simple saliva test for gluten intolerance. A good substitute for wheat is spelt, which is widely used in Europe for those with gluten intolerance and chronic disease. Spelt is a very nutritious and good-tasting grain.

Golden Grains High-Energy Breakfast Recipes

Grind dry, whole grains in an electric blender or a grain grinder to desired fineness. A very fine powder can be used as flour or a fast-cooking cereal. Coarser grinds give more fiber, texture, and variety. Experiment with different grains and combinations of grains. Combining different grains gives variety in flavor and nutrition. Combine grains with nuts and seeds to provide a good balance of amino acids. The ideal is to premix your grains and grind them just before cooking each day. If this is too time-consuming, try grinding enough for the week. Store the ground grains immediately in the refrigerator and cook fresh each morning. This is second best as far as freshness. A third alternative is to cook enough cereal for several days and reheat it each day. However, you get better flavor and nutrition by cooking grains fresh daily. These recipes make delicious breakfasts. Invent your own recipes, too!

SMOOTH OATMEAL CEREAL

1. Add ⅓ cup medium ground whole oats to 1 cup cold water.
2. Bring to a boil, stirring frequently. Then turn heat down to a low flame. Cover and let simmer 10 to 15 minutes.
3. Turn off heat and let the grains sit covered for a few more minutes.
4. Serve in a bowl.
5. Add 1 teaspoon to 1 tablespoon of raw, organic honey or maple syrup.
6. Pour a glass of sweet, edible-grade whey over the cereal for a breakfast that will also feed and promote the growth of your acidophilus colon flora.

MAKES 1 SERVING.

CREAM OF RICE CEREAL

1. Add ⅓ cup ground, long-grain brown rice to 2 cups cold water.
2. Bring to a boil, stirring frequently. Then turn heat down to a low flame. Cover and let simmer 10 to 15 minutes.
3. Turn off heat and let the grains sit covered for a few more minutes.
4. Serve in a bowl.
5. Add 1 teaspoon to 1 tablespoon of raw, organic honey or maple syrup.

6. Pour a glass of sweet, edible-grade whey over the cereal for a breakfast that will also feed and promote the growth of your acidophilus colon flora.

MAKES 1 SERVING.

GOLDEN ELIXIR CEREAL

This cereal has a good balance of carbohydrates and amino acid proteins.

1. Grind to a fine texture equal parts of the ingredients listed below. If you have a good grinder, it will be able to handle the softer grains like oats along with the tougher corn and oily nuts and seeds. In this case, you can put the whole mixture through the grinder at once. The blender will do a decent job. Otherwise, you can put your grains through the grinder and the nuts and seeds in the blender or a nut or coffee grinder. Grind this blend to a fine consistency for best taste and cooking.

Amaranth	Rye
Oats	Sunflower seeds
Almonds	Corn
Sesame and/or	Spelt
black sesame seeds	Pumpkin seeds
Barley	Chia seeds

2. Add ½ cup mixture to 1 cup water. (Experiment with amount of water to your desired taste.)
3. Bring to a boil, stirring frequently. As soon as it comes

to a boil, turn heat off. Cover and let sit for 5 to 10 minutes.
4. Serve in a bowl.
5. Add 1 teaspoon to 1 tablespoon of raw, organic honey or maple syrup.
6. Pour a glass of sweet, edible-grade whey over the cereal for a breakfast that will also feed and promote the growth of your acidophilus colon flora.

MAKES 1 SERVING.

GOLDEN PANCAKES

½ cup freshly ground pastry wheat flour
½ cup freshly ground oat flour
1 teaspoon cinnamon
1 tablespoon baking powder, aluminum-free
1 pinch sea salt
1 egg, slightly beaten
1 cup filtered water mixed with 3 to 5 tablespoons sweet, edible-grade whey

Grind whole pastry wheat and whole hulled oats in the blender or grain grinder to a fine consistency flour. Sift dry ingredients into a bowl.

Alternately add eggs and whey liquid to the dry ingredients, gently mixing together. Let mixture stand for a few minutes while the griddle heats up. Cook pancakes on the griddle and turn when golden brown.

MAKES 2 SERVINGS.

KAMUT PANCAKES

Follow the recipe above, but substitute ½ cup kamut flour for half of flour mixture.

Questions and Answers

Q. *What is the difference between soluble and insoluble fiber?*

A. Insoluble fiber is the indigestible fiber found in vegetables and whole grains. These insoluble fibers, naturally occurring in whole foods, contribute to colon health in several ways. They act as an intestinal broom, giving bulk and softness to the stool and assisting in the movement of feces through the colon. They help to give proper muscle tone to the muscular colon wall owing to the slight stretching of the wall from the bulk.

Persons with certain conditions, such as Crohn's disease, are unable to tolerate high-fiber foods owing to a loss of elasticity of the colon wall, which then becomes irritated and painful with any expansion.

Soluble fiber will dissolve in water and is found in fruits, legumes, and in grains such as oats. The primary action of soluble fiber is to delay the emptying time of the stomach, which assists blood sugar problems. Soluble fiber is especially noted for its action in helping to lower cholesterol in the body.

Q. *If fiber is so good for me, should I include fiber products like wheat bran or oat bran in my diet?*

A. Bran products are unnecessary and can cause problems in many people due to excess use. The best source of fiber is to eat the whole foods like vegetables and whole grains. Eating bran products is similar to eating sawdust. Bran is a processed food with very little nutrient content.

Since it is so dry, a person eating bran must consume large amounts of liquid to help push it through the system. Failure to do so can result in sluggish digestion and elimination. By including an abundance of vegetables and whole grains in your diet, you will provide ample amounts of naturally occurring bran fiber in a manner that your body can utilize effectively without causing problems.

Q. *But isn't bran supposed to be the best food for colon health?*
A. Naturally occurring fiber found in whole foods provides nutrients and helps the colon in various ways. However, bran fiber alone does nothing to promote colon health as it does nothing to help acidify the colon and does not provide food for the acidophilus flora. It's the flora, not the fiber, that's important to consider. As mentioned previously, the best way to help your colon health is through ingesting edible-grade sweet whey, to keep the colon acidified and the acidophilus bacteria thriving.

Q. *Why do I seem to get constipated when I take fiber like psyllium or bran? I thought they were supposed to act as laxatives.*
A. Psyllium expands to forty times its weight in water. When added to the already full colon, it can contribute to impactions. Bran is indigestible, dry fiber that can cause constipation in many people. A person consuming bran or psyllium may have a floating stool, but not a normal acidic colon pH.[1] A good test is to stop consuming these for a few days to a week and observe if the stool floats. If the colon is at its normal, slightly acid pH, large quantities of fiber (other than dietary fiber from whole grains and vegetables) may not be necessary.

SUMMARY

■

Many natural approaches to healing imbalances in the human body are available. The missing link in all health modalities today is the scientifically based reestablishment of the protective acidophilus colon flora as the foundation of proper elimination, health, and immunity. Our healthy acidophilus colon flora protects the body from invasive, pathogenic bacteria by producing a slightly acid colon pH and produces B vitamins and other nutrients that are utilized by the human host.

Our colon health depends primarily upon five factors:

1. Nutritious, whole food diet
2. Good digestion
3. A slightly acid pH in the colon
4. A predominantly acidophilus colon flora
5. Regular elimination

Most people today have either a deficient or depleted acidophilus colon flora owing to the use of antibiotics and other prescription medicines, use of street drugs, overuse of alcohol, poor diet, and continual exposure to pesticides, pollution, additives, and stress. Oral ingestion of acidophilus supplements is ineffective at recolonizing the colon primarily because they will not survive the strong stomach acids or high alkaline environment of the small intestine. Even if many acidophilus bacteria do reach the colon through the digestive tract, they will be overwhelmed by the commonly alkaline state of the colon.

Many people have acidophilus still latent in their colon whose growth and multiplication can be stimulated through good nutrition and the addition of edible-grade sweet whey to their daily diet. Sweet dairy whey is a nutrient-rich food which is the golden essence of milk. It contains no fat and is high in lactose (milk sugar), minerals, immunoglobulins, amino acids, and other nutrients specifically required by the protective acidophilus bacteria. Transformation of the colon flora can be accomplished within 4 to 8 weeks if the acidophilus flora is deficient and simply needs to be restimulated.

If the protective flora has been depleted, rectal replacement measures are needed. In these cases, the colon should be addressed directly through the rectal route by use of the WIT™.

Whey should be included in the daily diet throughout your life to feed and maintain the protective acidophilus flora. ProFlora™ Whey is the only whey *I* have seen beneficial results with in over twenty years of experience. Use of whey is the most important factor influencing colon health because it acidifies the colon and provides specific nutrients required by acidophilus. Other factors influencing colon health are good nutrition and diet to ensure optimal digestion and assimilation of nutrients, exercise to promote colon muscle tone and peristalsis, and a healthy lifestyle.

The colon flora functions as part of the immune system

by protecting the body from invasion by disease-forming bacteria and by supplying nutrients that contribute to human health. Research shows that when pathogenic bacteria predominate in the colon flora, metabolic by-products are produced that lead to inflammatory conditions, chronic degenerative diseases, and cancer.

When the colon and other organs of elimination are clear, elimination of toxins from the body is efficient and there is no reabsorption of toxins into the bloodstream. Products absorbed from the colon enter the portal vein to travel to the liver. Since the liver receives 70 percent of its blood from the portal vein, clearing the colon relieves any unnecessary toxic burden on the liver.

All living organisms depend on proper balance of the microecosystem for survival. Health practitioners today are concerned with reestablishing the health of the liver, lungs, and digestive and immune systems. When the colon is left in an alkaline state, it will adversely affect the health of the liver, lungs, digestive and immune systems—in fact, the entire body. To date, other than in this book, there has been little accurate information on either the role of the colon in health and immunity, the true definition of a healthy colon, or how to effectively achieve colon health. This book clearly shows that the colon is the soil of the body, providing our foundation of health, immunity, and longevity.

APPENDIX A

WIT™ PROGRAM RECOMMENDED PRODUCTS

■

"I have used the following products extensively with consistent, excellent results for over a decade. Because I am interested in positive, effective results for my clients, I can only recommend the products that I know work based on my experience."

—David Webster, founder Webster Implant Technique™

All of the following products are available from:

Advanced Health Solutions, LLC
PO Box 937
Cardiff by the Sea, CA 92007
1-800-943-0054 (call for free catalog)
www.uncom.com/colonhealth

ProFlora™ Natural Sweet Whey

Superior quality sweet whey that is delicious, light and fluffy. Classified as "edible" whey by the U.S. Department of Agriculture (USDA) which means it is made especially for human consumption. Instantly mixes in hot or cold water. This is the natural whey to feed and maintain your beneficial colon acidophilus flora. This is not a whey protein isolate. It is a whole foods whey, with naturally occurring minerals and amino acids and high in lactose, the milk sugar that acidophilus thrive on.

Kyo-Dophilus®

Highest quality acidophilus product on the market that I have found. Human-source acidophilus in a potent high-count culture necessary for successful colonization and lasting results. In my experience, the best way to use this product is for a rectal implant according to the Webster Implant Technique™. It is heat-stable and does not need refrigeration until it is opened.

Kyo-dophilus® is the only acidophilus product I have found that meets all the requirements of quality and has the research to prove it. They have been growing strains of human acidophilus for many years and include the most important strains of *L. acidophilus* and *B. bifidum* in their product. It is the only product I have used for rectal implants and seen lasting results within my clinical experience with over 3000 clients.

Kyolic®

Organically grown, odorless, aged liquid garlic extract. There are more than 150 published papers on the health benefits of Kyolic®, the original garlic extract. I recommend the liquid extract in the 2-ounce, red-label bottle. Because of the special, natural aging process, Kyolic® garlic does not irritate the acidophilus flora. Kyolic®'s unique aging process has resulted in over 235 peer-reviewed, scientific studies and research papers. The research done with Kyolic® has included liver protection, heart disease, cell protection, intestinal flora, removal of heavy metals, and allergies.

Kyo-Green®

Kyo-Green® is a special blend of greens that is well-balanced. It contains barley grass powder, wheat grass powder, Bulgarian chlorella, cooked brown rice and Pacific kelp. This blend of concentrated chlorophyll and high mineral plants cleans the blood and liver, enhances immune function and provides nourishment for the body. It has been found in studies to enhance immune function when 1 teaspoon is taken per day.

Genuine N-Zimes™

Plant enzymes that assist digestion of fat, starch, protein, and cellulose. Developed by enzyme researcher Dr. Edward Howell. These are the best quality digestive enzymes you will find. Dr. Howell found that plants create enzymes that help break food down into very small particles, allowing for better assimilation of nutrients.

American Whey by Jarrow Formulas™

All natural, biologically active protein isolate. Supports muscle development. Best source of clean, pure protein. Excellent for vegetarian diets. Add to smoothies with Pro-Flora™ Whey.

BioSil by Jarrow Formulas™

Biologically active silicon for bones, joints, hair, skin and nails. This product is from Belgium and has been thoroughly researched.

WIT KIT™

Most people are able to transform their colon flora to normal by using ProFlora™ Whey orally as part of their daily diet. However, some people may not have any latent acidophilus in their colons and so drinking whey will not be sufficient. For those with depleted colon flora, a self-help kit is available. Contains all the products and items you need, including an enema kit, to perform the Webster Implant Technique™ at home. Includes 17 pages of complete instructions and answers. You will not be able to do this procedure correctly without these full instructions. Follow the simple steps outlined in the instructions to help yourself achieve colon health. Once the acidophilus flora is reestablished, including ProFlora™ Whey in the diet will keep them thriving.

I receive many calls at my office from people who are unable to fly to California for the procedure. In response, I developed the WIT KIT™ which is a self-help version of my protocol. By carefully following the simple but detailed instructions, people can usually reacidify their colons and reestablish the acidophilus flora at home. It is essential to follow the instructions precisely or results will not be obtained. Furthermore, anyone with a health condition should consult their physician before using the WIT KIT™ since this protocol is a preventive measure and does not treat or cure any disease.

APPENDIX B

OTHER EXCELLENT PRODUCTS

■

Acidophilus
Available from the following company:

Wakunaga of America, Inc.
23501 Madero
Mission Viejo, CA 92691
Phone: 1-800-421-2998
PRODUCT NAME: Kyo-Dophilus® Capsules
Each capsule contains 1.5 billion cells of *L. acidophilus, B. bifidum,* and *B. longum.*

Drinking Water Systems
Available from the following company:

Multi-Pure Corporation
9351 Deerind Avenue
Chatsworth, CA 91313-4179
1-800-622-9206 (give ID number 105185)
They offer several excellent water filter systems that have been independently certified by the National Sanitation Foundation. Multi-Pure™ Drinking Water Systems remove

heavy metals, many pesticides, *Cryptosporidium, Giardia* cysts and chlorine from drinking water. Call or write for more information on their counter-top or under-the-counter filters or their whole-house system. I have used this system for over fifteen years.

Garlic
Available from the following company:

Wakunaga of America, Inc.
Phone: 1-800-421-2998
Makers of Kyolic®, Kyolic®-EPA and other supplements containing Aged Garlic Extract™ from organically grown garlic.

Grain Mills
Available from the following companies:

Millennium Outfitters, LLC
P.O. Box 51
Butte Falls, OR 97522
Phone: 541-865-3370
They carry the Country Living Grain Mill, one of the best quality grain mills available. Grinds the full range from coarse, cracked grains to fine flour. Attachment available to make nut butters and bean flours. They also carry food dehydrators, water filters, sprouting trays and other Country Living products. Write or call for their free catalog.

Champion Juicer with Grain Grinder Attachment
Great basic grain grinder. The juicer also makes nut butters. Available in most healthfood stores.

Green Drink (powdered source of vitamins, minerals and chlorophyll)

Available from the following company:

Wakunaga of America, Inc.
1-800-421-2998
PRODUCT NAME: Kyo-Green®
A combination of organically grown barley and wheat grasses, kelp, chlorella and brown rice. Two teaspoons provide the nutrients of a serving of deep green leafy vegetables.

Liver Supplements and Herbs

Available from the following companies:

Herb Pharm
1-800-348-4372
PRODUCT NAME: Dandelion and Milk Thistle Compound
This tincture contains a blend of quality herbs to support, cleanse and nourish the liver. Tinctures are liquid concentrates of herbs that have been extracted in alcohol (the amount of alcohol in a dose is minute). Since a tincture is liquid, it is absorbed very quickly into the system through the bloodstream since it does not undergo digestion. Available at health food stores.

Source Naturals®
23 Janis Way
Scotts Valley, CA 96066
Phone: 831-438-1144
PRODUCT NAME: Liver Guard

Unique antioxidant formula containing vitamins, minerals and antioxidants with herbs to target the liver and help improve its function. Available at health food stores.

PRODUCT NAME: Life Force Multiple without Iron
Excellent multiple focused on liver care and protection. Available at health food stores.

Mail Order
Available from the following companies:

Goldmine Natural Food Company
1-800-475-3663
Wide selection of hard-to-find organic grains, beans and seeds, wheat-free pastas, soy products, sea products and Japanese green teas.

Jaffe Brothers
P.O. Box 636
Valley Center, CA 92082
Phone: 760-749-1133
Top quality organic grains, nuts, seeds, virgin olive oil and more. All are kept in a refrigerated warehouse and shipped via UPS. Call or write for a catalog.

N.E.E.D.S.
Nutritional, Ecological & Environmental Delivery System
1-800-683-9640
Wide selection of supplements and vitamins, health and beauty aids, and books.

Misc. Supplements (vitamins, minerals, etc.)

Reliable and effective supplements are available from the following companies:

Carlson® Laboratories
15 College Drive
Arlington Heights, IL 60004-1985
Phone: 1-800-323-4141

Jarrow Formulas, Inc.™
1824 South Robertson Blvd.
Los Angeles, CA 90035-4317
Phone: 1-800-726-0886

Solgar Vitamin & Herb
500 Willow Tree Road
Leonia, NJ 07605
Phone: 1-800-645-2246

Source Naturals®
23 Janis Way
Scotts Valley, CA 96066
Phone: 831-438-1144

Natural Dairy Products

Available from the following companies:

Alta-Dena Dairy
Phone: 1-800-535-1369
Their milk has no pesticides, antibiotics or hormones. Distributed nationally.

Horizon Foods
Consumer Hot Line: 1-888-494-3020
Organic butter, milk and yogurt

Brown Cow Yogurt
Phone: 925-757-9209
Natural yogurt

Nancy's Yogurt
Phone: 541-689-2981
The original natural yogurt. The *L. acidophilus* and *B. bifidus* cultures are added after the yogurt is pasteurized, ensuring their viability.

Natural Meat Products (from free-range animals)
Available from the following companies:

Frontier Buffalo Company
Phone: 1-888-EATBUFF

Mannings
Phone: 1-800-283-2851

Natural Oil Products
Available from the following companies:

Barlean's
Phone: 1-800-445-3529
Excellent quality omega-3 oils, cold-pressed by a special method approved by Johanna Budwig, a German physician who developed the use of flax oil as a therapeutic method. These oils are pressed and kept refrigerated to ensure

freshness. They offer both flax oil and flax oil with borage oil.

Spectrum Natural Oils
Phone: 1-800-995-2705
High-quality line of salad and cooking oils, pressed using superior methods which preserve the nutritional value and flavor.

Vitamin E
Available from the following company:

Carlson®
1-800-323-4141
PRODUCT NAME: E-Gems®
Available in 30-1200 i.u. soft gels.

ORGANIZATIONS

■

AMERICAN ASSOCIATION OF ORIENTAL
   MEDICINE (AAOM)
433 Front Street
Catasauqua, PA 18032-2506
Phone: 1-888-500-7999
Fax: 610-433-1832

Call or write for a referral to a Licensed Acupuncturist
in your area. Oriental Medicine uses acupuncture, herbal
medicine, and other modalities to restore a person's
immune function and energy, and to facilitate the body's
healing processes and mechanisms. It is a useful adjunct
to proper colon care.

CANDIDA & DYSBIOSIS INFORMATION FOUNDATION
P.O. Drawer JF
College Station, TX 77841-5146
Phone: 409-694-8687

A private, nonprofit health organization created for the
purposes of public education and patient support services
and for data collection on chronic illnesses suspected of

having a fungal/mycotoxin etiology. A special emphasis is given to conditions characterized by an imbalanced intestinal microflora ecology. A referral list of M.D.s and other health care professionals who deal with these syndromes is available. Call or write for more information.

THE CENTERS FOR DISEASE CONTROL (CDC)
Phone: 404-332-4555
http://www.cdc.gov

Consumer information. Web site hosts up-to-date information on prevalent diseases and current infections.

LA LECHE LEAGUE INTERNATIONAL
1400 Meacham Road
P.O. Box 4079
Schaumberg, IL 60168-4079
Phone: 1-800-525-3243

Nationwide organization, established in 1956, that offers practical and reliable information on breastfeeding.

NATIONAL SANITATION FOUNDATION (NSF)
P.O. Box 130140
Ann Arbor, MI 48113-0140
Phone: 1-800-673-6275
Fax: 313-769-0109
http://www.ns8.org

An independent, not-for-profit organization of scientists, engineers, educators and analysts. NSF has served as a neutral agency in the areas of public health and the environment since 1944. One of its services is to evaluate, test and inspect drinking water treatment systems. It certifies products that meet NSF standards and conducts unannounced audits at the manufacturing plants of these devices to ensure maintenance of NSF standards. For a complete listing of NSF certified water filter systems, request the booklet, *NSF Listings—Drinking Water Treatment Units.*

APPENDIX D

RECOMMENDED READING

■

Dunne LJ. *Nutrition Almanac*. McGraw-Hill Publishing Company, New York, 1990.

Erasmus U. *Fats That Heal, Fats That Kill*. Alive Books, Burnaby, BC, Canada, 1993.

Erdmann R, Jones M. *Fats That Can Save Your Life: The Critical Role of Fats and Oils in Health and Disease*. Progressive Health Publishing, Encinitas, CA, 1995.

Gittleman, AL. *Guess What Came to Dinner: Parasites and Your Health*. Avery Publishing Group, Inc., Wayne, NJ, 1993.

Howell E. *Enzyme Nutrition: The Food Enzyme Concept*. Avery Publishing Group, Inc., Wayne, NJ, 1985.

Lau B. *Garlic and You: The Modern Medicine*. Apple Publishing Company Ltd., Vancouver BC, Canada, 1997.

Lau B. *Garlic for Health*. Lotus Light Publications, Wilmot, WI, 1988.

Levy SB. *The Antibiotic Paradox: How Miracle Drugs Are Destroying the Miracle*. Plenum Press, New York, 1992.

Life, Death and the Immune System. *Scientific American,* 1993.

Pitchford P. *Healing with Whole Foods: Oriental Traditions and Modern Nutrition.* North Atlantic Books, Berkeley, CA, 1993.

Rombauer IS, Becker MR. *Joy of Cooking.* The Bobbs-Merrill Company, Inc., New York, 1975.

Tierra M. *The Way of Herbs.* Pocket Books, New York, 1990.

NOTES

—

Introduction

1. Thomas CL. *Taber's Cyclopedic Medical Dictionary*. 18th edition. FA Davis Company, Philadelphia, 1997, 1420.

Chapter 1. The Fathers of Colon Health

1. Empringham J. *Invisible Friends of the Body*. Health Education Society, Los Angeles, CA, 1944:14–15.
2. Empringham, op. cit., 30.
3. Barghoorn ES. Colonic Therapy: Its Relation to Medical Practice. *The American Journal of Physical Therapy*. February 1932;8:304–306.
4. Hughens HV. A Bio-Physiotherapeutic Procedure in the Treatment of Non-Malignant Diseases of the Colon. *United States Naval Medical Bulletin*. May 1925;XXII(5):511.

Chapter 2. In the Beginning

1. Brock TD, Madigan MT. *Biology of Microorganisms*. 6th edition. Prentice-Hall, Englewood Cliffs, NJ, 1991:393.
2. Donaldson RM. Normal Bacterial Populations of the

Intestine and Their Relation to Intestinal Function. *The New England Journal of Medicine.* 1964;270(18):941.

3. Haenel H. Human Normal and Abnormal Gastrointestinal Flora. *The American Journal of Clinical Nutrition.* 1970; 23(11):1433.

4. Drasar BS and Hill MJ. *Human Intestinal Flora.* Academic Press, 1974:235.

5. Mackowiak PA. The Normal Microbial Flora. *The New England Journal of Medicine.* July 8, 1982; 307(2):83–93.

6. Jawetz E, Melnick JL, Adelberg EA. *Review of Medical Microbiology.* 16th edition. Lange Medical Publications, Los Altos, CA, 1984:293.

7. Lappe M. *When Antibiotics FAIL: Restoring the Ecology of the Body.* North Atlantic Books, Berkeley, CA, 1986:50–51.

8. Hamilton E. The Lost Art of Breast-Feeding. *Women's Times.* San Diego, CA, September 1993;33–34.

9. Wilson NW, Hamburger RN. Allergy to Cow's Milk in the First Year of Life and Its Prevention. *Annals of Allergy.* November 1988;61(5):323–327.

10. Hamilton, op. cit.

11. Sassen ML, et al. Breast Feeding and Acute Otitis Media. *American Journal of Otolaryngology.* September-October 1994;15(5):351–357.

12. Gilliland, SE, Speck ML. Antagonistic Action of *Lactobacillus acidophilus* Towards Intestinal and Foodborne Pathogens in Associative Cultures. *Journal of Food Preparation.* December 1977;40(12):820–823.

Chapter 3. Colon Flora: Our Protective Shield
1. Snyder RG, Traeger CH, Fineman S, Zoll CA. Colonic Stasis in Chronic Arthritis. *Archives of Physical Therapy, X-Ray, Radium.* October 1939;14:610–617.

2. Hibben JS. Irrigation of the Colon. *Archives of Physical Therapy*. 1940;21:33–40.

3. Traut EF. The Gastrointestinal Tract in Chronic Rheumatism. *Archives of Physical Therapy*. 1934;15:479–482.

4. Fishbaugh EC. Colon Disease and Its Therapy in Relation to Chronic Arthritis. *Archives of Physical Therapy*. July 1939;20:411–416.

5. Gibson GR, Roberfroid MB. Dietary Modulation of the Human Colonic Microbiota: Introducing the Concept of Prebiotics. *Journal of Nutrition*. 1995;125:1401–1412.

6. Seeley RR, Stephens TD, Tate P. *Anatomy and Physiology*. Times Mirror/Mosby College Publishing, St. Louis, MO, 1989.

7. Miller MA, Drakontides AB, Leavell LC. *Kimber-Gray-Stackpole's Anatomy and Physiology*. 17th edition. Macmillan Publishing Co. Inc, New York, 1977.

8. Thomas CL. *Taber's Cyclopedic Medical Dictionary*. 17th edition. FA Davis Company, Philadelphia, 1993.

9. Wrong OM, Edwards CJ, Chadwick VS. *The Large Intestine: Its Role in Mammalian Nutrition and Homeostasis*. John Wiley & Sons, 1981:173.

10. Joklik WK, Willett HP. *Zinsser Microbiology*. 16th edition. Appleton-Century-Crofts, New York, 1976.

11. Thomas CL. *Taber's Cyclopedic Medical Dictionary*. 13th edition. FA Davis Company, Philadelphia, 1977.

12. Seeley, Stephens, Tate, op. cit.

13. Donaldson RM. Normal Bacterial Population of the Intestine and Their Relation to Intestinal Function. *The New England Journal of Medicine*. April 30, 1964; 939.

14. Canon PR, McNease B. Factors Controlling Intestinal Bacteria: The Influence of Hydrogen-Ion Concentration on Bacterial Types. *The Journal of Infectious Diseases*. 1923;32:175–180.

Chapter 4. Defense Betrayed: Protective Shield Destroyed

1. Bergson MH. Effects of Bioisolation. *The American Journal of Clinical Nutrition*. 1970;23:1525–1533.
2. Pelczar MJJ, Reid RD. *Microbiology*. 2d edition. McGraw-Hill Book Company, New York, 1965:331.
3. Ibid., 331.
4. "Silver" Tooth Fillings Are Implicated in the Spread of Antibiotic Resistant Bacteria—An Increasing Problem in Medicine Today. The University of Calgary, Alberta, Canada. Press Release, April 1, 1993.
5. Levy SB. *The Antibiotic Paradox: How Miracle Drugs Are Destroying the Miracle*. Plenum Press, New York, 1992:114.

Chapter 5. The Toxic Colon

1. Gall LS. Normal Fecal Flora of Man. *The American Journal of Clinical Nutrition*. 1970;23:1457–1465.
2. Immerman A. Evidence for Intestinal Toxemia, An Inescapable Clinical Phenomenon. *The American Chiropractic Association Journal of Chiropractic*. April 1979; 13 (S-25):1-19.
3. Young G, Krasner RI, Yudkofsky PL. Interactions of Oral Strains of *Candida Albicans* and *Lactobacilli*. *Journal of Bacteriology*. 1956; 72(4):528.
4. Wyngaarden JB, Smith JLH, Bennett JC. *Cecil Textbook of Medicine*. 19th edition. WB Saunders Company, Philadelphia, PA, 1988:1898–1901.
5. Ibid., 1898–1899.
6. Fatalities Attributed to Entering Manure Waste Pits—Minnesota, 1992. *Morbidity and Mortality Weekly Report*. May 7, 1993;42(17):325–329.
7. Immerman, op. cit.
8. Drasar S, Hill MJ. Intestinal Bacteria and Cancer. *The*

American Journal of Clinical Nutrition. December 1972;25:1399–1404.

9. Newmark HL, Lupton JR. Determinants and Consequences of Colonic Luminal pH: Implications for Colon Cancer. *Nutrition and Cancer.* 1990;14(3–4): 161–173.

10. Malhotra SL. Faecal Urobilinogen Levels and pH of Stools in Population Groups with Different Incidence of Cancer of the Colon, and Their Possible Role in Aetiology. *Journal of the Royal Society of Medicine.* September 1982;75.

11. Hill MJ, Goddard P, Williams REO. Gut Bacteria and Aetiology of Cancer of the Breast. *The Lancet.* August 28, 1971;472–473.

12. Drasar, Hill, op. cit.

13. Hill, Goddard, Williams, op. cit.

14. Drasar, Hill, op. cit.

15. Javitt NB, Budai K, Miller DG, Cahan AC, Raju U, Levitz M. Breast-Gut Connection: Origin of Chenodeoxycholic Acid in Breast Cyst Fluid. *The Lancet.* March 12, 1994;343:633–634.

16. Finegold SM, Attebery HR, Sutter VL. Effect of Diet on Human Fecal Flora: Comparison of Japanese and American Diets. *The American Journal of Clinical Nutrition.* December 1974;27:1456–1469.

17. Gorbach SL. Estrogens, Breast Cancer, and Intestinal Flora. *Reviews of Infectious Diseases.* March–April 1984;6, Supplement 1.

18. Drasar, Hill, op. cit.

19. Finegold, Attebery, Sutter, op. cit.

20. Lee JR. *Natural Progesterone: The Multiple Roles of a Remarkable Hormone.* BLL Publishing, Sebastopol, CA, 1993.

21. Hill, Goddard, Williams, op. cit.

22. Drasar, Hill, op. cit.

23. Javitt et al., op. cit.

24. Finegold, Attebery, Sutter, op. cit.

25. Hill, Goddard, Williams, op. cit.

26. Aries VC, Crowther JS, Drasar BS, Hill MJ, Ellis FR. The Effect of a Strict Vegetarian Diet on the Faecal Flora and Faecal Steroid Concentration. *Journal of Pathology*. 1971; 103:54–56.

27. Javitt et al., op. cit.

28. Hill, Goddard, Williams, op. cit.

29. Drasar, Hill, op. cit.

30. Cummings JH, Hill MJ, Jenkins DJA, Pearson JR, Wiggins HS. Changes in Fecal Composition and Colonic Function Due to Cereal Fiber. *American Journal of Clinical Nutrition*. 1976;29:1468–1473.

31. Finegold, Attebery, Sutter, op. cit.

32. Walker ARP, Walker BF, Walker AJ. Faecal pH, Dietary Fibre Intake, and Proneness to Colon Cancer in Four South African Populations. *British Journal of Cancer*. 1986;53:489–495.

33. Donaldson RM. Normal Bacterial Populations of the Intestine and Their Relation to Intestinal Function. *The New England Journal of Medicine*. 1964;270(18): 938–945.

34. Maier BR, Flynn MA, Burton GC, Tsutakawa RK, Hentges DJ. Effects of a High-Beef Diet on Bowel Flora: A Preliminary Report. *American Journal of Clinical Nutrition*. 1974; 27:1456–1469.

35. Cummings et al., op cit.

36. Finegold, Attebery, Sutter, op. cit.

37. Lau B. *Garlic and You: The Modern Medicine*. Apple Publishing Company Ltd. Vancouver BC, Canada, 1997:96–97.

38. Ibid.

Chapter 6. Keys to Health: Colon and Liver

1. Guyton AC, Hall JE. Textbook of Medical Physiology. 9th edition. WB Saunders Company, Philadelphia, 1996:889.
2. Ibid., 877.
3. Brown L, ed. *The New Shorter Oxford English Dictionary.* Thumb Index Edition. Clarendon Press, Oxford, England, 1993.
4. Thomas CL. *Taber's Cyclopedic Medical Dictionary.* 17th edition. FA Davis Company, Philadelphia, 1993.
5. Spiro HM. *Clinical Gastroenterology.* 4th edition. McGraw-Hill, Inc., New York, 1993:415.
6. Seeley RR, Stephens TD, Tate P. *Anatomy and Physiology.* Times Mirror/Mosby College Publishing, St. Louis, MO, 1989.
7. Bland JS. A Functional Approach to Mental Illness— A New Paradigm for Managing Brain Biochemical Disturbances. *Townsend Letter for Doctors.* Reprinted with permission from *The Journal of Orthomolecular Medicine.* December 1994:1336.
8. Barral J-P. *Visceral Manipulation II.* Eastland Press, Seattle, WA, 1989:99.
9. Guyton, Hall, op. cit., 885.
10. Miller MA, Drakontides AB, Leavell LC. *Kimber-Gray-Stackpole's Anatomy and Physiology.* 17th edition. Macmillan Publishing Company, Inc., New York, 1977.
11. Thomas, op. cit.
12. Seeley, Stephens, Tate, op. cit., 635.
13. Rhoades R, Pflanzer R. *Human Physiology.* 2d edition. Saunders College Publishing, Philadelphia, 1992.
14. Guyton, Hall, op. cit., 885.
15. Lau B. *Garlic and You: The Modern Medicine.* Apple Publishing Company Ltd., Vancouver, BC, Canada, 1997:37–39.
16. Guyton, Hall, op. cit., 884.

Chapter 7. Organs of Elimination

1. Bland JS. A Functional Approach to Mental Illness— A New Paradigm for Managing Brain Biochemical Disturbances. *Townsend Letter for Doctors*. Reprinted with permission from *The Journal of Orthomolecular Medicine*. December 1994:1336.

2. Leviton R. Profile: Leon Chaitow. *East West*. September/October 1991;21(8):44–46.

3. Bland, op. cit.

4. Leviton, op. cit., 44–46.

5. Bland, op. cit.

6. Yanick P. Functional Correlates of pH in Accelerated Molecular and Tissue Aging. *Townsend Letter for Doctors*. May 1995;34–38.

7. Brown L, ed. *The New Shorter Oxford English Dictionary*. Thumb Index Edition. Clarendon Press, Oxford, England, 1993.

8. Empringham J. *Gland Reactivation and the New Knowledge of the Body*. Health Education Society, Los Angeles, CA, 1940:161.

9. Ibid., 145.

10. Stoy D, et. al. Cholesterol-Lowering Effects of Ready-to-Eat Cereal Containing Psyllium. *Journal of the American Dietetic Association*. 1993;93(8):910–911.

11. Damrau F. The Value of Bentonite for Diarrhea. *Medical Annals of the District of Columbia*. June 1961;30(6).

Chapter 8. Aging and Mental Health: The Colon Connection

1. Empringham J. *Invisible Friends of the Body*. Health Education Society, Los Angeles, CA, 1944:301–303.

2. Empringham J. *Intestinal Gardening for the Prolongation of Youth*. Revised and reprinted with new chapters.

Health Education Society, Los Angeles, CA, 1941: 11–17.

3. Mitsuoka T. Intestinal Flora and Aging. *Nutrition Reviews*. December 1992;50:438–446.

4. Empringham J. *Intestinal Gardening*, op. cit., 18–19.

5. Kaiser NW. Colonic Therapy in Mental Disease. *The Ohio State Medical Journal*. June 1930;26:510.

6. Ibid.

7. Ibid.

8. Bland JS. A Functional Approach to Mental Illness— A New Paradigm for Managing Brain Biochemical Disturbances. *Townsend Letter for Doctors*. Reprinted with permission from *The Journal of Orthomolecular Medicine*. December 1994; 1335–1341.

9. Ibid., 1336.

Chapter 9. The Missing Link: Setting the Record Straight

1. Goldin BR, Gorbach SL. The Effect of Milk and Lactobacillus Feeding on Human Intestinal Bacterial Enzyme Activity. *The American Journal of Clinical Nutrition*. May 1984;39:756–761.

2. Ibid.

3. Sneath PHA, Mair NS, Sharpe ME, Holt JG. *Bergey's Manual® of Systematic Bacteriology*. Volume 2. Williams & Wilkins, Baltimore, MD, 1986:1217.

4. Ibid.

5. Webster D. *Intestinal Gardening: Excerpts of Dr. James Empringham*. M.C. Winchester Publisher, Hermosa Beach, CA, 1986:21.

6. Mackowiak PA. The Normal Microbial Flora. *The New England Journal of Medicine*. July 8, 1982;307(2):88.

7. Ibid.

8. Friedenwald J, Morrison S. The History of the Enema

with Some Notes on Related Procedures, Part I. *Bulletin of History of Medicine.* 1940; 77–79.

9. Ibid.

10. Ibid., 91.

11. Ricci N, Caselli, M. Rectal Infusion of Bacterial Preparations for Intestinal Disorders. *The Lancet.* December 24/31, 1983;1494–1495.

12. Shahani KM, Ayebo, AD. Role of Dietary Lactobacilli in Gastro-intestinal Microecology. *The American Journal of Clinical Nutrition.* November 1980;33:2445–2457.

13. Bergson MH. Effects of Bioisolation. *The American Journal of Clinical Nutrition.* 1970; 23:1525–2533.

Chapter 10. Feed Your Acidophilus with Whey!

1. *Lactic Acid Bacteria in Beverages and Food,* op. cit.

2. *Handbook of Nonprescription Drugs.* 10th edition. American Pharmaceutical Association, Washington DC, 1993.

3. Davis JG. The Microbiology of Yoghourt. In: Carr JG, Cutting CV, Whiting GC, eds. *Fourth Long Ashton Symposium.* Long Ashton Research Station, University of Bristol, Academic Press, September 1973:19–21.

4. McDonough O, Alford O, Womack O. Whey Protein as a Milk Extender. *Journal of Dairy Science.* 1976; 59:34–40.

5. Thomas CL. *Taber's Cyclopedic Medical Dictionary.* 17th edition. FA Davis Company, Philadelphia, 1993.

6. Leibovitz B. Whey Protein: A Unique Source of Protein. *Muscular Development Magazine,* 1989.

7. National Academy of Sciences. *Improvement of Protein Nutriture.* Committee on Amino Acids, Food and Nutrition Board, National Research Council, Washington, DC, 1974.

8. Leibovitz, op. cit.

9. Brody T. *Nutritional Biochemistry*. Academic Press, San Diego, CA, 1994.
10. *Manual of Clinical Microbiology*. 5th edition. 1995:619.
11. *Handbook of Nonprescription Drugs*. 10th edition. American Pharmaceutical Association, Washington DC, 1993.
12. Morris GB, Porter RL, Meyer KF. The Bacteriologic Analysis of the Fecal Flora of Children with Notes on the Changes Produced by a Carbohydrate Diet. *The Journal of Infectious Diseases*. 1919;25:376.

Chapter 11. Nutrition, Lifestyle, and Colon Health

1. *Lactic Acid Bacteria in Beverages and Food,* Proceedings of a Symposium Held at Long Ashton Research Station, University of Bristol, September 19–21, 1973, edited by Carr, Cutting and Whiting, Academic Press.
2. Goldin B, Swenson L, Dwyer J, Sexton, Gorbach SL. Effect of Diet and *Lactobacillus Acidophilus* Supplements on Human Fecal Bacterial Enzymes. *Journal of the National Cancer Institute*. February 1980;64(2)255–261.
3. Drasar S, Hill MJ. Intestinal Bacteria and Cancer. *The American Journal of Clinical Nutrition*. December 1972;25:1399– 1404.
4. Hill MJ, Aries VC. Faecal Steroid Composition and Its Relationship to Cancer of the Large Bowel. *Journal of Pathology*. 1971;104:129–139.
5. Howell E. *Enzyme Nutrition: The Food Enzyme Concept*. Avery Publishing Group, Inc., Wayne, NJ, 1985.
6. EPA Finds High Lead Levels Across Nation. *Nutrition Week,* May 21, 1993.
7. Marchesani RB. *Cryptosporidium* Outbreak Hits Milwaukee: Seven Deaths Linked to Contaminated Water. *Infectious Disease News*. May 1993;6(5):1.
8. Hill MJ, Goddard P, Williams REO. Gut Bacteria and

Aetiology of Cancer of the Breast. *The Lancet.* August 28, 1971;472–473.

9. Drasar, Hill MJ, op. cit.

10. Cummings JH, Hill MJ, Jenkins DJA, Pearson JR, Wiggins HS. Changes in Fecal Composition and Colonic Function Due to Cereal Fiber. *American Journal of Clinical Nutrition.* 1976;29:1468–1473.

11. Finegold SM, Attebery HR, Sutter VL. Effect of Diet on Human Fecal Flora: Comparison of Japanese and American diets. *The American Journal of Clinical Nutrition.* December 1974;27:1456–1469.

12. Hill, Goddard, Williams, op. cit.

13. Drasar, Hill, op. cit.

14. Maier BR, Flynn MA, Burton GC, Tsutakawa RK, Hentges, RK. Effects of a High-Beef Diet on Bowel Flora: A Preliminary Report. *American Journal of Clinical Nutrition.* 1974; 27:1456–1469.

15. Erasmus U. *Fats That Heal, Fats That Kill.* 2d edition. Alive Books, Burnaby, BC, Canada, 1993.

16. Budwig DJ. *Flax Oil as a True Aid Against Arthritis, Heart Infarction, Cancer and Other Diseases.* Apple Publishing Company, Vancouver, BC, Canada, 1992.

17. Erdmann R, Jones M. *Fats That Can Save Your Life: The Critical Role of Fats and Oils in Health and Disease.* Progressive Health Publishing, Encinitas, CA, 1995.

Chapter 12. Golden Grains

1. Drasar BS, Jenkins DJA, Cummings JH. The Influence of a Diet Rich in Wheat Fibre on the Human Faecal Flora. *Journal of Medical Microbiology.* 1976; 9:423–431.

Index

ABOUT THE AUTHOR

David Webster is a best-selling health author and internationally known researcher and speaker on his specialty of colon health. Over the past twenty-two years he has compiled one hundred years of data from America, Europe, and Japan and discovered the missing link in health care today: the reestablishment of a healthy, slightly acid colon pH to harbor the beneficial acidophilus flora.

Acidophilus & Colon Health has been a best-selling basic book in health food stores since it first came out in 1980. This new updated version offers a definitive report that reveals the important role of the colon flora in immune function and health in more detail.

David is the originator of Webster Implant Technique™ (WIT), an effective method of colon hygiene based on his research and experience. He has eight years of clinical experience with WIT, which he offers in Encinitas, California, and has been educating people on how to reestablish their normal colon pH and flora since 1978.

David Webster offers a unique approach to health, combining microbiological facts with sound principles of colon health. He is here to set the record straight in the area of colon health, separating the many popular myths from the scientific facts.